A HEADACHE IN THE PELVIS

"One gloomy 5 a.m. in the winter of 2006, unable to sleep and trawling the Net yet again for some explanation of the chronic condition that had made my life a misery, I came across an extract from a book with the ugly title *A Headache in the Pelvis*. Here, after two years of expensive consultations and invasive medical tests, I found at last an accurate description of my plight.

"The authors David Wise and Rodney Anderson listed twenty-three symptoms, which would tend, they said, 'to take on a life of their own.' I had sixteen of them, including back pain, constantly changing abdominal pain, frequent nocturnal urination, and fierce twinges in legs and perineum. They called it chronic pelvic pain syndrome and concluded: 'The effects on a person's life have been likened to those of heart attack, angina, or Crohn's disease. Sufferers tend to live lives of quiet desperation. Anxiety, depression, and "catastrophic thinking" are the norm.'

"I was hugely cheered on reading this. . . . For two years I had oscillated between the conviction that I had cancer, or that my condition was psychosomatic. . . . As each medical test indicated that I didn't have cancer, I expected I'd quickly feel better. I didn't. . . .

"What to do? I had given up on official medicine. Its drugs made me sick. Its operations threatened my manhood without promising relief. . . . Now *A Headache in the Pelvis* talked about years of stressful overachieving, sitting at a desk, and an embattled mental attitude that had led me to tense the muscles of my pelvic floor so that they had atrophied and were pinching the nerves that crossed them from bladder, penis, and prostate. . . . I was definitely suffering enough. And growing curious. On your back, allowing your breath to establish its own pattern, eliminating all words from your mind, you focus on tension in the body and just, well, nothing, let it be. You go to meet the pain itself, and again, let it be.

"It took many months. . . . I shall remember for the rest of my life the day when, from the dry, knitted tension of my forehead, a great warm wave rose up and crashed across my chest and limbs, sweeping everything before it: thought, tension, pain. For five minutes I was pain free, utterly relaxed. It was the beginning of the way back."

—Tim Parks for the *London Times*

"This is a book that helps patients empower themselves in their own healing. With this book, patients learn how to gain control over their chronic pelvic pain. It is not a hocus-pocus solution; it is a long-term program that must be adapted into one's daily routine. I have witnessed firsthand how patients willing to change their behavior have been able to find healing. . . . When I see patients after they've read the book I can often see a change in their faces. To understand that we have the ability to affect our own healing process can be life changing."

—Ragi Doggweiler, MD, associate professor, director of Neuro-Urology and Integrative Medicine, Division of Urology, University of Tennessee, Knoxville

"After reading over the sixth edition of *A Headache in the Pelvis,* all I can say is 'Wow.' . . . Drs. Wise and Anderson have done it again! This has truly become the 'Bible' for patients, both men and women, who suffer from pelvic floor muscle dysfunction. The book demystifies a condition that is so frequently overlooked and often mistreated in clinical practice. It empowers patients to be their own caregiver, while it encourages partnerships with clinicians who can be tremendously helpful in the patient's path to symptom improvement.
    "*A Headache in the Pelvis* is on the top of my recommendation list."

—Robert Moldwin, MD, author of *The Interstitial Cystitis Survival Guide*

"Many pelvic pain patients go from doctor to doctor, specialist to specialist, without improvement, often feeling abandoned. A majority of patients with chronic pelvic pain do not respond to conventional therapies (antibiotics and anti-inflammatory drugs), leaving a huge void. Drs. Wise and Anderson offer a therapeutic option that can bring relief to many."

—Bart Gershbein, MD, clinical instructor, Department of Urology, University of California School of Medicine, San Francisco

"The sixth edition of *A Headache in the Pelvis,* by Drs. Rodney Anderson and David Wise, continues to be one of the most useful books for people who suffer from chronic pelvic floor pain. The book details a method for resolving pelvic pain by rehabilitating the pelvic floor muscles that have often been the brunt of anxiety or a reaction to a trauma or surgery. This new edition has filled in many of the answers raised since the publication of the first edition of this book in 2003. . . . This new treatment model is based upon Drs. Rodney Anderson and David Wise's work at Stanford University Medical Center."

—Erik Peper, PhD, professor, Institute of Holistic Health Studies, San Francisco State University

"Drs. Wise and Anderson have updated their important book on pelvic pain. This work has changed the way I think about pelvic pain. I now can find the clues in the physical exam (pelvic muscle spasm) that I had previously missed. This book is required reading for any clinician dealing with pelvic pain patients."

—Stephen Bearg, MD, obstetrician-gynecologist, past chairman, Department of Obstetrics and Gynecology, Marin General Hospital, Kentfield, California

A Headache in the Pelvis is an excellent book, brimming with warmth, compassion, and insight. It describes a pioneering method that empowers patients with pelvic pain to understand and help reduce their pain and symptoms. It is the very best kind of medicine, in that it teaches patients how to reduce their own symptoms themselves. This book is for people affected by pelvic pain and for family members who care about them; it's also for the medical providers who work with these patients."

—Marlene Cresci Cohen, PhD, director, Behavioral Sciences, Valley Family Medicine Residency, Modesto, California, and professor, Volunteer Faculty Department of Family Medicine, University of California, Davis

A Headache in the Pelvis is a lamp in the dark human suffering of chronic pelvic pain. This book is a precious document that will help many people."

—Robert Blum, MD, former chief, Department of Neurosurgery, Marin General Hospital, Marin County, California

"I highly recommend this book to colleagues, clients, and friends all the time. It does a great job explaining the connections between muscle tension and pain symptoms. . . . I find that after the first reading, the book needs to be read and reread."

—Marilyn Freedman, PT, DPT, BCB-PMD, CAPP

"This compelling understanding of chronic pelvic pain syndromes offers a new and pioneering approach to its alleviation."

—Frank Werblin, PhD, professor of neuroscience, University of California, Berkeley

"Since its first edition, *A Headache in the Pelvis* has been enthusiastically welcomed by patients suffering from urological pelvic pain syndromes (UCPPS), which may have been previously diagnosed as prostatitis or interstitial cystitis/painful bladder syndrome.

"I have specialized in UCPPS for over fifteen years and have been impressed by the educational merits of this book, which provides factual medical information to the patient without exacerbating fears or anxieties. Indeed, I have witnessed the therapeutic benefits of this book, as it provides validation to patients along with empowering management strategies. *A Headache in the Pelvis* addresses both the physical and emotional aspects of UCPPS in a caring and methodical way, which patients find accessible and nurturing. It has become a wonderful adjuvant to physiotherapy and self-care, as well as a support tool for loved ones living with a man or woman who has UCPPS.

"Although I recommend *A Headache in the Pelvis* to all of my patients, I have happily discovered that more and more physical therapists are recommending the book to their referring doctors and to their patients. In many ways, this book communicates effectively to a wide audience, as it is accessible and empowering to patients, interesting and insightful to health care providers."

—Jeannette Potts, MD, director, Center for Pelvic Pain, Alternative and Medical Urology Services, Urological Institute University Hospitals of Cleveland, Case Western Reserve University

"*A Headache in the Pelvis* is a very important contribution to understanding and treating pelvic pain. It is also an illuminating discussion of the relationship of mental and physical interaction in the production of disease and an approach to a truly comprehensive treatment of illness that has relevance to a whole range of contemporary morbidities."

—Donald L. Fink, MD, professor emeritus, University of California, San Francisco School of Medicine

"The work described here by Drs. Wise and Anderson is at the forefront of the understanding and treatment of chronic pelvic pain syndromes like prostatitis. Their approach sees the big picture of these disorders and breaks new ground in our understanding of the subtlety of the mind-body continuum."

—A. S. Hadland, MD, former director, Integrative Medicine Pain Management Service, Kaiser Permanente

"It is important for the patient to learn all he can about his disease, especially if he has prostatitis/chronic pelvic pain syndrome. That is difficult because doctors seldom agree on the cause, cure, or treatment. The information contained in *A Headache in the Pelvis* will be essential for these patients."

—Mike Hennenfent, president of the Prostatitis Foundation

"This book is something different, something not seen before in the field of prostatitis/chronic pelvic pain. This book will take you to a place you have never been before within prostatitis/chronic pelvic pain syndrome. The relaxation techniques, exercise, and trigger point release all are outlined and explained in great detail. Examples used to explain various points are truly excellent and enlightening. Pick up this book and you will be taken into a world of relaxation, calm, and above all a way to possibly ease your symptoms. The authors have created a new portal into the condition and offer you through the book just what they do to help sufferers get better. Lie back, relax, and you will not be able to put this book down. To suddenly be aware of your pelvic pain in the ways outlined in this book is a truly enlightening experience. This time last year we could not have dreamed it possible to see a book like this on the bookshelf.

"One of the authors of this book tells you about his own twenty-two-year struggle (which he won) with chronic pelvic pain syndrome ('a headache in the pelvis') so it's from a sufferer's perspective. At times you will often say to yourself YES, I feel like that, when reading this book and smile simply because you will feel one thing: the authors understand my problem. Every UK urologist should read this book. If you can afford it, you may wish to buy your doctor a copy."

—The British Prostatitis Support Association

A HEADACHE IN THE PELVIS

The Wise-Anderson Protocol
for Healing Pelvic Pain

THE DEFINITIVE EDITION

DAVID WISE, Ph.D.,
RODNEY ANDERSON, M.D.

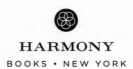

HARMONY
BOOKS · NEW YORK

Many readers have found that reading this book has helped them better deal with or reduce their symptoms. This book, however, is not intended as a stand-alone self-help book and is not meant to be a substitute for competent medical or psychological or physical therapy, diagnosis, instruction, or supervision in home self-treatment. The aim of the *Wise-Anderson Protocol* is to help patients become independent and to be able to reduce or resolve their symptoms themselves without reliance on others. This independence requires training with and consultation by those competent in *Extended Paradoxical Relaxation* and *Trigger Point Release*. Our approach is used when medical evaluation has ruled out physical illness and pathology.

Published in the United States by Harmony Books, an imprint of the Crown Publishing Group, a division of Penguin Random House LLC, New York.
crownpublishing.com

Harmony Books is a registered trademark, and the Circle colophon is a trademark of Penguin Random House LLC.

Library of Congress Cataloging-in-Publication Data has been applied for.

ISBN 978-1-5247-6204-9
Ebook ISBN 978-1-5247-6205-6

Printed in the United States of America

Cover background by ilolab/Shutterstock

10 9 8 7 6 5 4 3 2 1

First Edition

*This book is dedicated
to the many brave men and women
who suffer daily from pelvic pain.*

CONTENTS

A PERSONAL NOTE FROM DR. WISE

After suffering from pelvic pain and dysfunction for twenty-two years, I conducted a very long and personal research into the subject on a mission to heal myself. Today, I am grateful to have been symptom-free for years.

During the first several years without pain, I was reluctant to share what I'd discovered. In addition to being reticent to talk about pelvic pain publicly, I was superstitious that if I told my story, somehow the blessing of having no more pain would be taken away.

Over the years, I treated others with pelvic pain at Stanford and watched many of them improve, the kind of real improvement like my own that I rarely saw with any other treatment. I became more confident that the method that I used for my own recovery was substantial and should be communicated to people who were suffering as I had. My desire to help those with nowhere to turn overcame my embarrassment about sharing things most people don't share with others.

I am a psychologist. I contacted and joined with Dr. Rodney Anderson, the renowned neurourologist (a urologist specializing in the neurology of urologic disorders) at Stanford University Medical School, where he ran a chronic pelvic pain clinic. He had long been the court of last resort for many people with pelvic pain. I shared the method I used to resolve my pelvic pain with Dr. Anderson. After this meeting, I began working as a visiting research scholar with Dr. Anderson at Stanford University Medical Center in the Department of Urology with patients with pelvic pain. For eight years we pioneered the development of the treatment that became the *Wise-Anderson Protocol*. Later colleagues and I began offering treatment for pelvic pain in the form of a six-day intensive clinic which we have been doing approximately monthly, and continue to do up to the present moment. Dr. Anderson, I, and colleagues have published a number of articles in the *Journal of Urology* and other scientific journals on the results of our treatment. This book is the result of our collaboration.

During these early years, this protocol was presented at meetings for researchers at the National Institutes of Health, the American Urological Association, the American Physical Therapy Association, the International Continence Society, the Association for Applied Psychophysiology and Biofeedback, and other scientific meetings. In 2003, Dr. Anderson and I published the first edition of *A Headache in the Pelvis,* describing the protocol that we first used at Stanford over the past eight years. *A Headache in the Pelvis* has sold widely and been received enthusiastically. This definitive edition offers vital information to the many millions of individuals suffering from pelvic floor-related pain.

In 2003, after my time at Stanford, I began doing the protocol that Dr. Anderson and I developed at Stanford as a six-day immersion clinic in Sonoma County in California as a way of coordinating treatment and consolidating in one place. Patients continue to come from far away to learn the *Wise-Anderson Protocol* in the intensive immersion clinics and be trained to be able to do the protocol on a daily basis without the assistance of professionals.

Competence in self-treatment has turned out to be the most effective way the protocol can be used. The six-day immersion clinics that have continued to be offered on a monthly basis since 2003 up to the present are now not affiliated with Stanford. For years, Dr. Anderson continued to evaluate many patients at Stanford and refer them to the immersion clinic when they are appropriate candidates. From 2003 to the present, Rodney Anderson, physical therapist Tim Sawyer, and I have actively and enthusiastically collaborated in research on patients seen in the immersion clinics, held now in Santa Rosa, California.

Since 2005, we have published articles in the *Journal of Urology* and other journals on data from patients they have collaboratively seen and treated. I was a plenary speaker at the National Institutes of Health in 2005, presenting research on the *Wise-Anderson Protocol*. Dr. Anderson has presented research on this protocol at meetings of the American Urological Association and other professional meetings. The Internal Trigger Point Wand that I invented years ago is centrally used in the *Wise-Anderson Protocol* and is the only FDA-approved device for efficacy and safety and was given an award by the American Urological Association. Our new Trigger Point Genie that I also recently invented is an amazing tool for external trigger point release and is part of our protocol. Dr. Anderson, Tim Sawyer, and I continue to do research on patients to improve our treatment and deepen understanding of the healing of pelvic floor dysfunction.

When I see patients who describe the misery they are in because they are hurting constantly, I understand. For years, I was in continual pain. More times than I can remember, I would wake up in the middle of the night weeping because my pain was so great and I saw no solution.

The doctors whom I saw were in the dark about my condition and no one had any idea of what I was going through. There was no Internet at that time, no support groups, and little access to any information on my condition. I would go to the medical library at a local hospital, or the medical library at the University of California Medical Center, and pore over old medical journals looking for some kind of clue that might help me. Then, after what felt to me like a lifetime, through some serendipity, I found a way out. Below I share with the reader a little bit about my journey.

When I was twenty-eight years old, I remember sitting in my office and feeling an uncomfortable sensation in my rectum. I remember first thinking that perhaps I was sitting on something. I got up and looked and, lo and behold, there was nothing there. I came to describe this sensation as if a golf ball were lodged up inside and I could not get it out. No matter how I moved, what exercise I did or diet I tried, this feeling persisted. Along with rectal pain, I experienced the need to urinate frequently. To my dismay, my bladder never felt quite empty after urination. Intercourse sometimes was uncomfortable and often seemed to exacerbate my symptoms. Over the course of years I was symptomatic, I experienced almost every symptom we discuss in this book.

I went to see a urologist, who gave me both good and bad news. The good news was that he couldn't find anything wrong. There was no infection, no growth or abnormality in the prostate or surrounding area. The bad news was that he couldn't find anything wrong and therefore couldn't help me. He called what I had "prostatosis," which meant, I believed at the time, the discomfort and urinary frequency and urgency that I felt somehow came from the prostate gland, though the prostate gland was normal. The diagnosis actually didn't really make any sense to me, but I was too scared to ask more about what it meant. I now think the doctor didn't know what it meant either.

I was lucky to find a kind doctor. I say I was lucky after seeing many patients, some of whom saw doctors who did invasive procedures, surgeries, and put them on courses of antibiotics and medications for years that didn't help. The doctor whom I found was wise enough to recognize that he didn't know what was going on with me and didn't offer any heroic measures despite my suffering. So many doctors of the patients we have seen have "gone to school" on their patients with treatments that often made them worse.

I would see my doctor regularly, sometimes every three or six months. He would do a prostate exam, extract prostatic fluid, go into another room where he looked at the fluid under a microscope, and then come back into the little examination room I was in and say, "It is clear—no infection." I would ask him, "Is there anything new being tried, any new research?" He would reply: "No, not now, but I think this gets better as you get older and there is less sexual activity." That statement offered little consolation. My doctor believed that somehow there was something wrong with my prostate gland even though he couldn't find anything wrong with it. As I later found out, my doctor's misunderstanding was a misunderstanding of the doctors of many of our patients. To this day it still is.

My doctor's diagnosis was reassuring to me, however incorrect. I desperately needed to be reassured that somehow there was hope that I could get better. I noticed that the more anxious I was, the worse my symptoms got. As someone who tends toward anxiety, I think I would have had a more difficult time without this doctor's kind but inaccurate assurance.

I tried everything. I started out with the regular medical treatments of antibiotics, which did not help me. I experimented with diet, cutting out alcohol, coffee, and spicy foods on the advice of the physician I was seeing. There was no benefit. Someone told me that certain reflexology pressure points near the ankle could help. I pressed those pressure points to the point of great pain for many months hoping for some relief. I read somewhere that zinc deficiency could cause my problem, and so I took zinc supplements regularly. I tried many sessions of acupuncture, psychotherapy, guided imagery visualization, hands-on healing, and prayer. Nothing made a difference to my condition. I lived with pain and the failed interventions I tried for many years. This is why I deeply understand the plight of those who suffer with pelvic pain.

Indeed, nothing helped in any lasting way, whether the intervention came from my doctor or from my own research. While there was almost always an underlying sense of discomfort, when flare-ups would occur, often after sex, they would last for months and months. Many patients have asked me how I lived with these symptoms for twenty-two years. As I reflect now, there was no magic to it. I muddled through. Nothing heroic about this. It's just that there was no alternative in my mind to going on, from day to day. The cost to my quality of life was very high. I often found myself distracted and I withdrew inwardly from social situations and my loved ones. Miraculously, I never took off work, even though I very much understand how someone would. In the language of current-day America, "You do what you gotta do."

My symptoms waxed and waned, but never went away. After years of having symptoms, I found myself in the fortunate position of not having to work. I had dreamed about this for many years and somehow it became a reality.

The effect of my newfound freedom on my pelvic pain was not what I expected. It never occurred to me that my anxiety would increase. In fact, my symptoms got much worse when I retired. More than that, their severity became constant and I found no relief day or night. I remember well lying in bed during a heavy rainstorm. Being in a warm bed and hearing the rain on the roof had been one of my pleasures, but during this time there was no pleasure because I could find no escape from the constant aching that I felt.

In my desperation, I began making phone calls to doctors and researchers around the world whose names I took from the medical literature. It was from this desperate search that I discovered a way to stop my symptoms that developed into the basis of what is now called the *Wise-Anderson Protocol.*

After several months of using the protocol of my own crude version of trigger point release and relaxation described in this book, I occasionally did not feel the need to go to the bathroom for four or five hours. This felt amazing to me. As time went on, I would notice that I was pain-free for brief periods. These periods gradually increased. Later, weeks passed when I had no symptoms.

To my dismay, there were still many flare-ups and my symptoms would return full-blown. The flare-ups, however, lasted a fraction of the time that they used to. I was getting better. Imperceptibly, over a long time, my regular state became one of no pelvic pain or dysfunction.

I felt normal. I was grateful beyond words for the feeling that everything inside was working right. The joy of feeling normal in my bladder was beyond my ability to communicate. Feeling normal is a peculiar way to describe how I felt, because it really doesn't communicate the ease and pleasure I felt about something that most people never even notice and simply take for granted. And aside from close friends being happy that I was feeling good, my sense was that no one really understood how it felt inside me to simply feel normal.

It took well over two years for all of the symptoms to go away. To this day, I continue to use the relaxation protocol and I believe it has been essential in my remaining well.

I hope this book brings some clarity and direction to many who suffer from pelvic pain. It is written for those who have no familiarity with medical terminology or research.

David Wise, Ph.D.
San Francisco, California

A PERSONAL NOTE FROM
DR. ANDERSON

M any years ago I had the privilege and pleasure of being men-
tored by one of the giants of American urology. Dr. Thomas A.
Stamey, chairman of the department of urology at Stanford University,
introduced me as a resident in training to the problems that men endured
with chronic prostatitis. More important, he introduced me to a way of
evaluating patients with meticulous detail, being curious and mindful
of every nuance of symptom and finding. He reiterated continuously
the importance of paying attention to detail and being a "thinking"
urologist as opposed to mindlessly throwing pills at or cutting your way
through a problem. He also showed me through his clinical research
methods that it was much better to study a few patients thoroughly than
a lot of patients superficially.

Dr. Stamey taught me to look through the microscope and see what
human inflammatory cells looked like in the prostatic fluid of men suffering with prostatitis. He got quite excited to demonstrate fat-laden
macrophages that exhibited a Maltese-cross appearance under polarized
light. He showed me how to carefully segregate the urine specimens
from the prostatic fluid to prove whether a patient had true bacterial
colonization of the prostate or some contaminant. His publication with
our other colleague, Dr. Edwin Meares, still stands as the pivotal work
to define prostatic infection.

Unfortunately, no matter how much we have studied this problem
of chronic prostatitis and chronic pelvic pain syndrome, in both men

and women, three decades later we still do not understand why it happens and how to prevent it. Fortunately my partner Dr. David Wise, a perceptive psychologist, came along and described his experience and discoveries in abating his symptoms after having dealt with his condition for many years. Since that time I have been impressed that this approach helps many more people than pharmaceutical agents or surgery.

This book is our attempt to convey to the patients suffering from chronic pelvic pain syndromes our genuine concern for their well-being and to describe our experience with an alternative approach to improve or resolve their symptoms. At the same time we attempt to help clarify and explain the controversies and medical investigations ongoing to elucidate the biologic basis of these complaints.

Rodney U. Anderson, M.D., FACS
Stanford, California

CHAPTER 1

CHRONIC PELVIC PAIN IS EASY TO UNDERSTAND

Millions of men and women suffer from pelvic pain, discomfort, or dysfunction that drugs, surgery, and conventional treatment do not help. If you are one of them, you may have experienced rectal, genital, or abdominal discomfort or pain, increased discomfort or pain sitting down, discomfort or pain during or after sexual activity, or urinary frequency, urgency, and hesitancy.

If you're reading this book, you've probably gone to a doctor or many doctors who found little or no physical basis for your symptoms. Your tests came back normal. You may have been diagnosed with pelvic floor dysfunction, prostatitis, chronic pelvic pain syndrome, levator ani syndrome, pundendal neuralgia, coccydynia (tailbone pain), chronic proctalgia, proctalgia fugax, pelvic floor myalgia, piriformis syndrome, interstitial cystitis, urethral syndrome, or other related diagnoses, but found no relief. We are proposing in this book that all of these different diagnoses are essentially different names for the same problem, a problem we are calling *A Headache in the Pelvis*.

The amelioration or resolution to the kind of pelvic pain we treat and discuss in depth in this book has eluded the best medical minds for recorded history. Most people reading this book would not be reading it if they were able to find help within the context of conventional treatment. It is not uncommon for individuals with pelvic pain to either have it on a continual basis or to have it wax and wane for many years and to go from doctor to doctor receiving little help. To date, there is no solution to this problem offered by the best conventional medicine. Conventional or not, for the most part, there is very little that has helped pelvic floor–related pain and dysfunction. The *Wise-Anderson Protocol* offers real understanding and help.

Pelvic pain we describe is a condition of sore, irritated pelvic floor tissue that is never given a chance to heal. Our book offers an intimate understanding of this problem based on one of the author's twenty-two-year history with it and his experience of its resolution as well as a subsequent twenty-four years of experience of treating several thousand patients in collaboration with skilled colleagues. We discuss this understanding in detail in the next chapter. Instead of pelvic pain with related symptoms discussed in this book being the result of an infection, a trapped nerve, an autoimmune disorder, or degenerative disease, we propose that it is a psychophysical problem. Both the physical and psychological aspects must be directly addressed for any chance at a satisfactory resolution of symptoms.

AN INTIMATE LOOK AT PELVIC PAIN

The major contributing factor involves a chronically knotted up, contracted pelvis—typically a physical response to years of worry—that leads to tight, irritated pelvic floor tissue, leading to a reflex response in the pelvic tissue of protective guarding that creates a self-feeding cycle that gives pelvic pain a life of its own. In what we can call pelvic pain related to pelvic floor dysfunction, sore pelvic floor tissue once established doesn't have a chance to heal the way other sore human tissue heals. You can think about the ongoing reflex protective guarding of irritated, sore pelvic tissue as a kind of ongoing pelvic charley horse. This chronic charley horse keeps the pelvic tissue irritated and preventing its otherwise natural healing. Ongoing pain from this sore tissue leads to protective pelvic muscle guarding, anxiety, continued dysfunctional protective guarding, and chronic painful tissue irritation.

*In scientific studies, it has been documented
that the* Wise-Anderson Protocol
helps a majority of patients.

Dealing with these central aspects of pelvic pain is daunting in the most ideal of circumstances. With the best of treatment we can offer, resolving one's pelvic pain is a challenge and with some individuals beyond our ability to help. But we do help the large majority of those we treat. Indeed, the large majority of qualifying patients are helped by the program explained in this book, called the *Wise-Anderson Protocol*.

HOW THIS BOOK CAN HELP YOU

You are holding in your hands the seventh, definitive edition of *A Headache in the Pelvis*. It is a streamlined edition of a book that we originally published in 2003. Since its publication, the book has been read by tens of thousands, and the feedback from readers has informed our refinements to the protocol, as has our clinical work. Some readers of our book have reported that they have significantly reduced their symptoms by reading about and then applying the methods we describe here. That being said, we cannot recommend using the methods that we describe here on oneself or others without proper supervision from someone competent in these methods. We don't know how a reader relates to his or her body and do not want to be responsible for actions individuals take, in relationship to themselves, that we cannot supervise and correct when necessary. Pressing on a trigger point for one individual may mean using too little pressure, for another just enough pressure, and for another bruising pressure. The process described in *Extended Paradoxical Relaxation* may result in a significant relaxation of tension and symptoms in one individual, yet in another individual this instruction may be wholly misinterpreted and result in tension that increases and that sours him on using this method.

Nevertheless, some readers have designed their own programs using our model and have helped themselves. They have written to us with gratitude for our road map.

The basic goal of the *Wise-Anderson Protocol* is to train patients to become expert in reducing or stopping their own symptoms. We have found that when treatment for pelvic pain by a professional is confined to weekly or biweekly visits without a committed self-treatment daily program of pelvic floor relaxation, stretching, and effective physical therapy self-treatment, it tends to be a tepid intervention. The *Wise-Anderson Protocol* sees the treatment of pelvic pain as an inside job.

SELF-TREATMENT IS THE CORE OF OUR METHOD

For understandable reasons relating to constraints of time in conventional treatment, training patients in self-treatment tends to be an afterthought in most treatments of pelvic pain. Lip service is given to patient daily self-treatment but with little time for patient training or backup. The *Wise-Anderson Protocol* makes the training of the patients in doing their treatment its primary goal.

THE *WISE-ANDERSON PROTOCOL* IS NOT EASY OR QUICK

Most of us are resistant to changing our routine. It is our experience that taking at least two hours or more a day to do one's home program for at least many months is the bare minimum for our protocol to be effective. Carving out two hours or more from one's life bumps up against real barriers for most people. These barriers include the huge inertia of a routine shaped by the demands of work and family and a desire for downtime that often makes one feel there is no room for any other activity. Our patients tend to stick to their home practice over the long term when they see that their symptoms are improving.

In our experience, only the yearning to get out of pain and the related suffering of pelvic pain syndromes is a strong enough motivation for patients to accommodate the self-treatment requirements we describe.

A ROAD MAP OF PELVIC PAIN HEALING

The biggest contribution we have to offer *is a new view of the problem of pelvic pain and a road map for its amelioration.* If we have done this in writing this book, we have accomplished something important. However this book is used, we hope that the *Wise-Anderson Protocol* can shine a light on the path of resolving pelvic pain.

THE DIFFERENT NAMES FOR PELVIC PAIN: THE ELEPHANT AND THE BLIND MEN

Chronic pelvic pain goes by many names. You will find a comprehensive list in this chapter. It may be called *prostatitis* by a urologist or *coccygodynia* or *pudendal nerve compression syndrome* by a colorectal surgeon. Other names used to describe the same condition include *chronic genital pain, prostatodynia, pudendal neuralgia essential anorectal pain, idiopathic pelvic pain, pelvic floor dysfunction, pelvic floor myalgia, levator ani syndrome,* and *spastic piriformis syndrome.* Three specialists may give you three different diagnoses.

There's an old parable about ten blind men who came upon an elephant. One touched the elephant's leg and remarked, "Oh, this creature is like a tree trunk." Another was under the stomach, pushed up, and said, "Oh, no. This creature is like a soft ceiling." A third pulled the tail and said, "No, this creature is a rope connected to a tree." All the blind men were right and all the blind men were wrong; their answers were incomplete because they each had access to limited information. Similarly, there's a lack of communication among many medical specialists; if they all spoke to each other, they would see that they are often talking about the same condition. In this book, we aspire to see the whole elephant.

THE SOURCE OF PELVIC PAIN SYMPTOMS

There is a simple psychophysical basis for chronic pelvic pain symptoms. The seemingly wide array and variability of the symptoms are simply expressions of the same underlying problem, whether you're a man or a woman. The *Wise-Anderson Protocol* does not treat the symptoms; instead, it treats what triggers those symptoms. Our approach substantially reduces or abates symptoms in a large majority of qualifying patients who undertake our full protocol.

In this book we will use the terms *a headache in the pelvis, chronic pelvic pain syndrome(s), chronic pelvic pain, pelvic pain,* and *CPPS* synonymously to refer to all the conditions discussed.

DIAGNOSES YOU MAY HAVE RECEIVED

MEN
- Prostatitis (National Institutes of Health categories)
  I. Acute bacterial prostatitis
  II. Chronic bacterial prostatitis
  IIIA. CPPS nonbacterial inflammatory prostatitis
  III. CPPS nonbacterial noninflammatory prostatitis
  IV. Asymptomatic inflammatory prostatitis
- Orchalgia and/or epididymitis

WOMEN
- Urethral syndrome
- Vulvodynia (vulvar vestibulitis)

BOTH MEN AND WOMEN
- Pelvic floor dysfunction
- Interstitial cystitis
- Levator ani syndrome
- Pudendal nerve entrapment syndrome (pudendal neuralgia)
- Proctalgia fugax

THROUGHOUT HISTORY, PELVIC PAIN DISORDERS HAVE NEVER HAD A SOLUTION

For many years, chronic pelvic pain syndromes have posed an enigma to the medical/healing community. In men, nonbacterial prostatitis, for example, has routinely been confused with acute or chronic bacterial prostatitis, even though an accurate and easy method for diagnosis has been available for years. At the same time, nonbacterial prostatitis, which makes up the overwhelming number of cases of prostatitis, tends to be regarded by doctors as a kind of wastebasket diagnosis for pelvic symptoms that the doctor does not understand or know how to treat. Gross pathology, as measured by the latest medical instruments, has not been able to explain the degree of suffering caused by these disorders.

*Doctors often tell patients with chronic
pelvic pain syndromes that they can find
little or nothing wrong with them.*

What we are proposing in this book is that these conditions are rather like a headache, except that the location of the headache is in the pelvis. Hence *A Headache in the Pelvis* is our title. And the basis for all these conditions is chronic pelvic floor muscle irritation, triggered and perpetuated by chronic muscle tension. If chronic pelvic pain syndromes are, in fact, a headache in the pelvis, then treatment needs to be radically different from what has traditionally been followed.

A Headache in the Pelvis is the name we are giving to chronic pelvic pain syndromes where no gross pathology has been found. These syndromes involve pain, often pain and dysfunction related to urination, defecation, and sexual activity. This discomfort or pain and dysfunction occurs in both men and women. One person may experience only one symptom, while another may experience all symptoms. Sometimes symptoms inexplicably vary from day to day or week to week. Symptoms vary, as do their anatomical locations, yet we propose that the trigger for these symptoms is the same and that a common effective treatment exists for all of them.

Even though many people suffer from a headache in the pelvis, most of them feel alone in their difficulty. The pelvic area is considered private and is often very difficult to talk about, even with close friends or relatives. Basically, most people want the areas of the genitals and rectum to work but don't want to know much about them or to have to pay any attention to them.

These areas of the body are not treated with much appreciation. This is a truth that is reflected in how we word profanities. What do we call people with whom we are angry? Usually terms related to defecation or procreation. Indeed, these are terms of denigration. In our culture, the genitals and rectum are shrouded in shame and guilt. When a pelvis becomes chronically sore and irritated, sufferers often feel alone and afraid and are reluctant to share their experience, especially as they find neither a doctor nor a friend who can really understand their symptoms.

Quite simply, if you haven't experienced chronic pelvic floor pain and dysfunction, it's hard to understand it because you've never experienced the weird kinds of symptoms that occur with it. The healing of the abused pelvis, as Steven Levine has stated eloquently, in part involves bringing the genitals and rectum "back into the heart."

COMMON SYMPTOMS IN MEN AND WOMEN WITH PELVIC PAIN

Below is a list of the most common symptoms we see in the patients we have been able to help. Most experience several to many of the symptoms. Rarely do patients have all of them.

Urinary Symptoms: Frequency, Urgency, Hesitancy, Dribbling, Dysuria (Burning with Urination), Nocturia (Nighttime Urination)

Frequency and Urgency
- Urinary frequency in our patients ranges from annoying to debilitating.
- There is commonly a feeling of something always nagging in the bladder/urethra/genitals, and typically, after patients urinate, they report that they don't feel "emptied" during or after urination and are left with the feeling of having to urinate again even though there is little to urinate.
- Frequency/urgency can result in the feeling of having to be near a bathroom; sometimes one can hardly hold in the urge to urinate when it arises. Some patients feel that their lives revolve around staying near a toilet.

Nocturia (Frequent Nighttime Urination) for Men and Women
- Urinary urgency and frequency at night can deprive patients of sleep.
- Exhaustion from sleep deprivation tends to feed into the cycle of tension, pain, protective guarding, and anxiety.

Dysuria (Discomfort, Pain, or Burning Before, During, or After Urination)
- Discomfort, pain, or burning during urination is associated with pelvic-floor dysfunction.
- When the trigger points, chronic spasm, and myofascial contraction of the pelvic muscles are resolved, dysuria is also resolved in many of our patients.
- Some patients experience discomfort only after urination, not during.
- In a subset of individuals, dysuria can be quite painful, and urination becomes an ordeal and sets off further pain.

Reduced Urinary Stream and Hesitancy of Urination
- In men it is important to medically evaluate whether the reduced stream is caused by prostate enlargement or other issues.
- This symptom can be worsened when urine is held in longer than comfortable (because we speculate that the tightening of the muscles to hold in the urine can result in a kind of spasm that is slow to release upon urination).
- Reduced urinary stream can be a contributing symptom to low self-esteem and hypochondriasis, especially in our younger patients.
- When urinary symptoms are part of muscle-based chronic pelvic pain syndrome, we have found that the flow of urine can improve after the pelvic floor is loosened.

Sitting Pain
- Sitting can trigger or exacerbate pelvic discomfort/pain/symptoms.
- Sitting is one of the great sufferings in pelvic pain; it makes all aspects of normal life difficult and can lead to the fear that one may not be able to work.
- Sitting pain usually starts out mild in the morning, but after one has sat through the day there is increased discomfort that can last into the night.
- Sitting pain can make it difficult to fly or drive for any distance without aching.
- Some patients have to go on disability because sitting is a requirement of their jobs.

Perineal Discomfort (Pain Between Scrotum and Anus or Vagina and Anus)
- The perineum is one of the most common sites of pelvic pain, is intimate, can hurt 24/7, and may be very distressing. The perineum is the place where most muscles of the pelvic floor attach, has many sources of referred pain, and can be experienced on one side or another.

- The perineum is often the site of bicycle-riding pain.
- Perineal pain can be made worse by sitting or standing.
- In a 2009 Stanford study of our work published in the *Journal of Urology,* we documented that 79 percent of our patients complained of pain in the perineum.
- The perineum, the anal sphincter, and the tailbone are parts of the body where patients can experience the feeling of "sitting on a golf ball."

Discomfort or Relief After a Bowel Movement

- Relief after a bowel movement occurs when the tight pelvic muscles relax.
- Discomfort after a bowel movement can be particularly disconcerting if that post–bowel movement pain triggers symptoms more strongly for the rest of the day.
- Little is written about this symptom when it occurs in the absence of hemorrhoids or anal fissures, but in our experience it is common.
- The mechanism of defecation typically involves the filling up of the rectum with stool, which sends a signal for the internal anal sphincter and puborectalis muscle to relax and triggers the experience of urgency to have a bowel movement.
- Once the stool passes through the relaxed anal sphincter and out of the body, the internal anal sphincter reflexively closes.
- When someone has pelvic pain and exacerbation of symptoms after a bowel movement, we propose that the internal anal sphincter tends to "overclose"; we propose that the sphincter reflexively overtightens instead of resuming its normal, relaxed, resting tone.
- Sometimes patients experience a nagging urgency to have a bowel movement throughout the day even when they have little to evacuate.
- The overtightening of the internal sphincter typically can be felt digitally.

- Post–bowel movement pain appears to occur less frequently when someone is relaxed and not hurried, and whatever contributes to a more relaxed state during a visit to the bathroom may reduce this symptom.
- Resolving post–bowel movement pain in our patients tends to occur as their entire chronic pelvic muscle tension and irritability releases.

Genital Pain
- Women can commonly have pain inside the vagina, on one side or another.
- In women, vulvar pain sometimes accompanies pelvic pain.
- Some men have pain in the tip or shaft of the penis, often irritated when touched or rubbing against underwear.
- Not uncommonly, men can have slight redness and skin irritation at the tip of the penis.

Pain Above the Pubic Bone (Suprapubic Pain)
- Suprapubic pain is common with patients who have urinary frequency, urgency, hesitancy, and anterior symptoms.
- Sometimes pressing on this area can refer into the anorectal (anus and rectum) area, and bladder pain is sometimes experienced here as well.
- Pain can be on one side or another or in the middle.

Coccyx (Tailbone) Pain (Coccygodynia/Coccydynia)
- Tailbone pain is common. It is typically referred pain from the pelvic floor or muscles attached to the tailbone and is not from the tailbone itself.
- Some patients we have seen who had their tailbones removed typically felt no relief.

Coccygectomy (surgical removal of the tailbone) has typically failed to help anyone with pelvic pain.

- Coccyx pain is often related to post–bowel movement pain, sitting pain, and rectal pain.

Low Back Pain (on One Side or Both)
- Low back pain is common and often confuses patients and practitioners because the symptoms are referred from the muscles of the pelvic floor, not the low back.
- Discomfort can be on either side and can migrate from one side to the other.

Groin Pain (on One Side or Both)
- Groin pain is sometimes confused with the pain of a hernia.
- We have seen patients have hernia repair that did not resolve their groin pain.
- We have seen patients whose pain began with testicular, inguinal hernia or other surgeries. CT scans, MRIs, X-rays, blood tests, and other diagnostic tests typically fail to detect any problem in those with muscle-based pelvic pain. What is disconcerting to many patients with chronic pelvic pain syndromes is that conventional medical testing—including imaging, blood and urine tests, and other diagnostics—fails to document any abnormalities or point in any therapeutic direction. Conventional medical treatment—including antibiotics, alpha blockers, anti-inflammatories, analgesics, and all surgeries and procedures—typically shows little and points in no therapeutic direction.

Dyspareunia (Pain with Sexual Activity in Both Men and Women), Sexual Dysfunction
- Sexual activity can be painful either during or afterward.
- In women, pain is felt on the outside of the vagina, the inside, or both. Because there is often *vaginal pain* at the opening or inside the vagina, *dyspareunia* (pain during or after intercourse) is almost always present. In more severe cases, particularly with women who have *vulvar vestibulitis,* there is an *inability to have intercourse.* This may be their only complaint.

- In men, the area of the pelvic floor, the penis, and the base of the penis can hurt or feel tight, and sometimes pain can be experienced upon ejaculation; also, postejaculatory pain or discomfort can be experienced in the urinary tract. Some men report that their ejaculate no longer comes out strongly but rather dribbles out and/or that orgasms feel weaker or different. Sometimes patients have erectile dysfunction (occasional or frequent inability to attain or maintain an erection), softer erections, and reduced sexual pleasure.
- Sexual pain can lead to reversible sexual dysfunction, erectile dysfunction, reduction of libido, anxiety, and sex-related lowered self-esteem.
- Many patients suffer from reduction in intimacy related to difficulty with sexual activity.
- Pelvic examination in which trigger points are palpated can often re-create symptoms of pain felt during sex.

Reduced Libido (Reduced Interest in Sex)
- Reduced interest in sex is common with pelvic pain.
- In muscle-related pelvic pain, there is typically no pathology of the physical structures involved in sexual activity.
- Our view is that reduced libido is a mix of anxiety, reduced self-esteem, and pelvic pain. The resolution of pain and dysfunction of the pelvic muscles usually helps resolve reduced libido.

Depression
- For many patients who are in the throes of pelvic pain, the thought that it will never go away triggers depression.
- When doctors cannot help, and one sees no light at the end of the tunnel, depression or anxious depression is the rule rather than the exception.
- Depression involves the feeling of helplessness about changing what feels critically wrong in one's life.

Anxiety and Catastrophic Thinking (Projecting Catastrophe into the Future)
- The most difficult part of pelvic pain tends to be the catastrophic thought that it will never go away.
- Anxiety and catastrophic thinking distract patients' attention away from life, can paint an unacceptable picture of the future, and strongly arouse the nervous system, which in turn can increase pain.
- Pelvic pain typically occurs in individuals who tend to be anxious and catastrophize.

Social Withdrawal and Difficulty in Intimate Relations
- The withdrawal results from chronic pain and its ability to distract the person from any enjoyment of the moment.
- Chronic pelvic pain takes a major toll on relationships in that the pain makes it very difficult to be fully present and enjoy the company of one's partner, family, or friends.

Impairment of Self-Esteem
- Self-esteem almost always declines when one has pelvic pain.
- Men and women with chronic pelvic pain often worry that no one will want to be with them or that they will not get to do the things they wanted to do with their lives.

Sleep Disturbance
- Sleep disturbance is common.
- Patients who tend to wake up to urinate during the night, or wake because of pain and anxiety, are deprived of sleep because they have difficulty going back to sleep having once woken up in an aroused and distressed state.
- At Stanford, we published a paper about the precipitous rise in cortisol in the morning among pelvic pain patients.

Helplessness and Hopelessness

- Helplessness and hopelessness are the deepest suffering with chronic pelvic pain.
- Helplessness comes from a patient's inability to stop pain/discomfort that is draining and scary.
- Hopelessness in pelvic pain patients arises when they can't see anything on the horizon that might help them or change their current situation for the better.

Heat (Hot Bath or Shower, Heating Pad) Helps Temporarily

- Hot baths and/or heat temporarily reduce symptoms (when possible we recommend getting into a hot bath or hot tub as opposed to a "sitz bath").
- Less commonly, cold or ice helps.
- Cold weather can cause symptoms to flare up in some patients.

Benzodiazepines Temporarily Reduce Symptoms When First Used

- The family of drugs called benzodiazepines (Valium, Klonopin, Xanax, Ativan) can often relieve symptoms for a few hours and are helpful when used skillfully and not regularly.
- Benzodiazepines can be addictive, and they lose effectiveness when used for long periods of time.
- Benzodiazepines typically make the user feel tired and so should not be used when one is driving or has to be alert.

For both sexes, all of the symptoms can be either intermittent or constant and can be diurnal or nocturnal (daytime or nighttime). They can occur during sitting or standing, and are often more profound during periods of stress. Symptoms can involve discomfort or pain and no urinary or sexual dysfunction, discomfort or pain and urinary symptoms with no sexual symptoms, or both. One of the perplexing aspects is the variable cycles of intensity.

CHAPTER 2

UNDERSTANDING THE
WISE-ANDERSON PROTOCOL

It's not a good idea to do open heart surgery
if the problem is heartburn.
—Anonymous

The answer to an unsolved problem is rarely
found in the field designated to study it.
—Martin Schwartz, Ph.D.

THE WAY YOU SEE A PROBLEM
IS THE KEY TO SOLVING IT

Changing our ideas of disease alters the way we treat it. On an individual level, your notions about what is wrong with you determine what you will do to help yourself. In modern times we have discarded the idea that illness is caused by humors. None of us would consider bloodletting or purging to improve our health. It is equally important, however, to be clear today about the thoughts and assumptions we hold about pelvic pain that motivate our choice of treatment.

Fifty years ago, two gastroenterologists who did research at a medical center near New York conducted an experiment to show the effect of one's mental picture of a bodily condition on the condition itself. These researchers did rectal examinations of naive male subjects. Looking up the rectum of a subject, one of the two doctors present would casually say to the other, within earshot of the subject, that something looked cancerous inside the rectum. The other doctor would agree, and then they would observe what happened in the subject's colon. The researchers reported that commonly the colon of the subject would go into an immediate spasm. As soon as the doctors reassured the subject that he was healthy and did not have cancer, the spastic colon immediately released. This experiment illustrated how a catastrophic idea about your health can have an immediate and profound physical effect.

Fear typically makes symptoms worse. Hope and reassurance typically make them better.

Negative and catastrophic thinking palpably increase discomfort or pain in those diagnosed with pelvic pain. Many of the men we see with prostatitis are, at some level, worried they have cancer or some other life-threatening disease. It is not uncommon for patients with pelvic pain to walk around for many years carrying catastrophic thoughts relating to their pain that, as we will discuss later, exacerbate their pain and impoverish the quality of their lives. *The reassurance that what they have is not life threatening can even alleviate their symptoms on a short-term basis.*

THE POWER OF TRUST, REASSURANCE, AND THE PLACEBO EFFECT

A placebo is commonly thought of as a sugar pill, essentially a substance with no known medically active ingredient. It is thought that the power of the placebo derives from the patient's belief that the pill will help.

Most placebo medication is given during randomized controlled trials, and participating in the trials adds a huge amount of "placebo effect." It is a form of behavioral conditioning.

When you talk about the placebo effect, you are talking about the effect of feeling that "you are going to be okay." The placebo effect is the great antidote to anxiety and fear.

PLACEBO IS THE STRONGEST OF MEDICINE

Some have suggested that the placebo effect is the highest form of body-mind healing. Indeed, combining the placebo effect with the use of effective methods can only enhance the methods. The power of placebo attests to the power of a *thought* to reassure people that they are safe and that everything will be okay. The power of placebo indirectly attests to the power of fear to disturb both body and mind because placebo simply acts to remove fear and doubt.

This also appears to be the chief ingredient in the power of a good doctor's bedside manner. In the presence of such a doctor, the patient's anxiety dissolves in the idea that all will be well again. This is not unlike a child's trust that his loving parents will take care of him.

If you are experiencing pelvic pain or discomfort now and the anxiety and contraction that usually come with it, imagine that someone were to say to you, "We will take care of this. You will be completely healed and back to normal." Notice what effect this might have on your symptoms. Many people with pelvic pain experience a reduction or sometimes even an abatement in symptoms on a short-term basis as the result of trying something new that they think will help them. That placebos tend to temporarily help muscle-based pelvic pain supports the common observation that stress and mental factors play a significant role in the condition.

It is agreed among researchers in the field that there is a substantial placebo effect with *any* treatment for chronic pelvic pain. For example, antibiotics have become one of the reliable foundations of contemporary medical treatment. We all have a profound respect for antibiotics and their power. We believe however, that the short-term relief that people with a nonbacterial condition obtain from antibiotics is primarily borrowed from this huge public confidence and that, in the case of pelvic pain, it is a result of the placebo effect.

The power of placebo is not small. A dramatic example occurred with a man who had suffered from pelvic pain for ten years. He reported that he entered a doctor's office in a great deal of pain. The doctor, whom the patient described as kindly and confident, felt this patient's prostate gland and said, "Your prostate is completely normal. Our test revealed no evidence of anything wrong. Go out with your wife and have a night on the town and celebrate your good fortune." The man reported he left the doctor's office with no pain. Moreover, he remained pain-free for months, even though the pain gradually returned. There is no known medicine that can alleviate pelvic pain for months. This illustrates that the placebo effect and the trust that everything will be okay, on a short-term basis, have the ability to loosen the knot of chronic tension and anxiety that binds the contents of the pelvis.

Placebos work only as long as the person either consciously or unconsciously believes the problem has been solved. The difference between our treatment and a placebo is critical. As we shall discuss, we actively assist our patients, training them in what we call *Extended Paradoxical Relaxation* (EPR) without their having to hold on to any belief. In fact, the focus of EPR is to let go of attachment, from moment to moment, in any belief or thought. When a pelvic pain patient follows the instructions of EPR, the patient practices repetitively shifting attention away from the stream of thought that typically enthralls their attention to their subjective sensation of what is already relaxed inside them, and in this way the nervous system calms down and the irritated tissue continues its healing journey.

WHAT YOUR DOCTOR TELLS YOU HAS A HUGE EFFECT ON YOUR VIEW OF YOUR LIFE AND YOUR FUTURE RELATED TO YOUR CONDITION

In our culture, the doctor is thought to understand the true reality of the patient's mental and physical state. Typically, patients with pelvic pain adopt the doctor's viewpoint of their condition, and they adopt the implications of the diagnosis as well. The doctor's diagnosis can add to a sense of fear and foreboding that patients already carry with them. For example, a doctor's suggestion that prostatitis may be an autoimmune disorder, a suggestion that is simply theory with little data to support it, can easily scare patients who are already confused. Many doctors lose sight of how much their ideas communicate to patients. An offhand comment that a doctor makes to a patient can either haunt or relieve a patient for years.

A Stanford psychiatrist found that women with breast cancer who participated in support groups lived significantly longer than those who did not. This was startling information and demonstrated the profound positive impact of social/psychological factors in creating disease on the one hand and extending life and well-being on the other.

HOW YOU NAME WHAT IS WRONG WITH YOU CAN HURT YOUR CONDITION OR HELP IT

If the positive thought of knowing that there is a place to share your deepest feelings can enhance both the quality and length of life, as was the case in the Stanford study, so too can adverse thoughts injure you. A number of researchers have found that the *diagnosis* of cancer itself can traumatize individuals. Studies have shown that some people who have been diagnosed with cancer subsequently exhibit signs of post-traumatic stress disorder. These signs derive, not from the physical presence of cancer, but from the terror that the diagnosis triggers.

SOMETIMES THE DIAGNOSIS YOU ARE GIVEN IS MORE TRAUMATIZING THAN THE CONDITION ITSELF

It is not difficult to understand why the diagnosis of cancer is a traumatic event. Imagine what it would mean to your life if a doctor told you that you had cancer. Your life would inevitably change as the shock of the diagnosis settled in. Even if it was untrue and the doctor had made a mistake in his diagnosis, the diagnosis alone would shake you to your foundation. *What you call what is wrong with you can hurt you or help you.* Sometimes the diagnosis you are given is more traumatizing than the condition itself.

THE TERM *CHRONIC* USED TO DISCUSS PELVIC PAIN MAY BE MORE HURTFUL THAN HELPFUL

The term *chronic* means "ongoing and continual" and implies that the condition will not go away. If you are diagnosed with having chronic pelvic pain, you may believe that the condition will never go away. That's why we prefer the term *pelvic pain* or, better yet, *a headache in the pelvis,* a term that reflects our compassionate interest in discussing these difficult conditions in a credible way that does not condemn people to dismal future outcomes. Indeed, our title reflects our optimism for the possibility of a successful resolution of the problem.

LIMITATIONS OF THE TRADITIONAL MEDICAL MODEL: VIEWING THE LIMITATIONS OF SEEING YOUR BODY AS A MACHINE WITHOUT CONSCIOUSNESS

When we see a doctor, the nurse often puts us in a small, windowless room where we wait on an examining table or sit on a chair. We busy ourselves, often nervously, reading a magazine until we hear the door open and the doctor enters. He talks to us for a few minutes, perhaps examines our body, and then gives us a piece of paper, which we take to the pharmacy. When all goes well, and after a few pills, the complaint is resolved.

We take for granted that the doctor usually does not talk to us about our thoughts, feelings, home situation, sex life, or spiritual practices. We assume it is normal for the doctor to be interested only in the specific problem for which we are in the office, a problem with our body. Furthermore, we take for granted that the actual time spent with the doctor will probably be a few minutes or less.

We know that modern medicine typically looks at the body as a machine. However, the implications of that view are profound and far-reaching. If the body is a machine, it is a thing, an object, a piece of meat. The body, in some profound way, is not considered to be conscious, to have any intelligence, or to be something to which one has to listen carefully.

When the body is seen as a machine, one searches for the defective part to be fixed. An illustration of this is found in the treatment of vulvar vestibulitis. Doctors observe redness at the bottom of the vagina, which the woman reports as tender. For some physicians, the solution to this problem has been to surgically remove this red and irritated tissue. In our experience, the results have largely been ineffective.

One of the implicit assumptions in the treatment of muscle-based pelvic pain in the various conventional medical treatments for it in the past 50 years is that it is fundamentally a physical problem requiring a physical intervention. While lip service is sometimes made to the role of consciousness in the creation and perpetuation of the problem, the treatments offered almost exclusively address attempts to fix the physical body, without concern for someone's state of mind.

In our practice, we have seen patients whose prostates have been removed, whose pelvic muscles have been surgically severed, whose bladders have been removed, whose testicles have been removed, whose pelvic nerves have been dissected, and whose pelvic stabilizing ligaments have been severed—all in the service of getting rid of the part of the body/machine that is thought to be the source of the problem. The patients we have seen who have undergone such medical care have most often not been helped by such interventions, and more often have had to endure greater suffering, not only from the original source but from the surgical interventions.

The rest of the person, including his or her way of thinking, emotional state, lifestyle, values, and, importantly, causes of fear and anxiety—things that are not measurable—tends to have only secondary importance in the doctor's office. When the doctor examines the patient and can find no part of the body that appears to be causing the problem, the doctor often concludes that the problem is mental. To the patients we have seen, this kind of diagnosis has been invalidating and depressing, and the treatments they have undergone for the "mental" condition have routinely failed to help their problem.

In treating your painful pelvic floor from the current body-as-a-machine perspective, it is as if the doctor were saying to your pelvic floor: "You must have been invaded by bacteria or are inflamed for some reason. I am going to use drugs or do surgery to get rid of the bacteria or inflammation. Your pain is something that shouldn't be there. It is not informative. It shouldn't be considered or listened to, just gotten rid of."

When the doctor brings this viewpoint to the suffering of someone with a chronic pelvic pain syndrome, the patient often adopts the following kind of view of his or her own pelvic floor:

I feel your discomfort, burning, pain, tightness, soreness, or rawness, and I am afraid of you. The doctor wants to get rid of you but can't. He doesn't seem to know what's wrong with you. Whatever I try to do does not get rid of you. You might mean terrible things. You may mean that I can never have health, happiness, joy, love, relationship, parenting, and fulfillment in my life. You shouldn't be here. You are a mistake, an error, and a defect in me. You have nothing to say to me. You are bad.

Whenever I feel you, I feel afraid and discouraged. I want to get as far away from you as possible. I hate you and want to get rid of you.

YOUR BODY WANTS TO HEAL

The old medical model views the body as composed of modular parts that can be replaced or repaired when defective. This modular model seems to dismiss the notion that the body has intelligence and consciousness and that it can heal itself.

Dr. Dean Ornish pioneered a treatment that derives from a dynamic and functional way of understanding the body. He offered a treatment for individuals with heart disease that put them on a low-fat diet, taught them yoga, and provided them with group support. He discovered that when his patients followed this multifaceted regimen, the blocked state of their arteries reversed.

> *A painful pelvic floor does not want*
> *to be in pain, yet it doesn't have the*
> *words to tell you what it needs*
> *to be out of pain.*

Dr. Ornish demonstrated the truth that *the body has the intrinsic capability of regenerating and healing itself under the right conditions.* By *intrinsic,* we mean that this ability for regeneration and self-healing is part of the very nature of the body. In the healing process, the challenge is to learn how to provide the best environment for healing to occur.

Nowhere is the dynamic and intelligent nature of the body more visible than in the effects of exercise. Sit in a chair without moving for three or four weeks and your muscles atrophy. Your heart muscle will actually diminish in size because the requirement for pumping blood has been reduced. Those who have been bedridden for a prolonged period know all too well the effect of no exercise on muscle tone and strength and general well-being.

All of us have observed that when we cut ourselves, clean the wound, and put a Band-Aid over it, a miracle occurs. In a number of days, the cut is healed. Most of us take this miracle for granted and simply expect this stunning intelligence of the body to do its own healing. If a car that was damaged in a car accident could gradually fix a dent or scrape all by itself we would be stunned and regard this event as a miracle.

*Healing pelvic pain means understanding
and cooperating with what a painful
pelvis needs in order to heal.*

We know the cut does not need our conscious effort or direction to heal. The healing is intrinsic, natural, and in the very nature of tissue. There is, however, a condition necessary for the healing to occur. *One must give the cut an environment within which it can heal.* Pick at it, allow dirt and bacteria to enter it, and it won't heal. The key is to understand what the requirement for healing is and make it a reality. This is obvious for some conditions and not so obvious for other conditions. In the past, when human beings did not understand that microbes that were invisible to the eye could enter a wound and infect it, they often failed to make the kind of environment needed for their healing.

The current thinking by researchers in this area does not seem to be focused on making the pelvis whole, sound, and well. In our book, we are proposing that to treat pelvic pain and dysfunction one must first understand what the pelvis needs to become whole, sound, and well. *We are proposing that the key to healing in general and the resolution of certain kinds of pelvic pain and dysfunction in particular involves learning skills that will free the healing forces in the body.* And in general, helping muscle-based pelvic pain heal means releasing the chronic pelvic contraction and calming down the aroused nervous system that feeds the contraction and interferes with the healing of the sore and irritated pelvic tissue.

When you appreciate the intelligence of your body and see your symptoms as your body trying to talk to you, you take a different viewpoint from the one resulting from the conventional medical model. From this viewpoint, it is as if you are saying to your pelvic floor:

I feel your burning, pain, tightness, soreness, or rawness, and it doesn't feel good to me, and I know it doesn't feel good to you. I know you want to feel better and be out of pain. I know you are happiest when you function properly. I know that you wouldn't be complaining this way without a reason. I know you want to heal, to be whole, sound, and well. I want to understand what you are saying to me in your pain and dysfunction and listen to how I can help you. I care about you.

Such a viewpoint closes the separation between you and your pelvic floor. It brings an attitude of peace and understanding to your pain and dysfunction. It does not wage a war. Such an attitude relaxes and does not tighten. It sees the sore, contracted area of the pelvis as an inarticulate friend in need and not an enemy. It brings love, not hate; integration, not separation; and compassion and understanding, not fear.

The language of a painful pelvis can be difficult to decipher unless you listen carefully and want to understand its language.

WHAT YOUR PELVIC PAIN IS TRYING TO TELL YOU

You can think of muscle-based pelvic pain as caused by sore irritated pelvic tissue that triggers a reflex guarding in the pelvis that triggers a self-feeding cycle of tension, sore, painful pelvic tissue, anxiety and protective guarding. The state of reflex chronic guarding against the sore tissue containing pain-referring trigger points, reduced blood flow, and an inhospitable environment for the nerves, blood vessels, and structures throughout the pelvic basin that promotes pelvic muscle irritablity.

Understanding that the central feature of pelvic floor pain is uncomfortable/sore pelvic tissue irritated by chronic pelvic floor tightening that gives rise to reflex guarding against this sore tissue, anxiety about the discomfort that increases electrical activity in trigger points—*in short, a vicious cycle of sore pelvic tissue, triggering reflex pelvic muscle tightening, irritating the sore tissue, triggering anxiety, which increases pelvic tension and pain, increasing trigger point electrical activity, and triggering more guarding in the irritated tissue.*

This understanding has pointed us in the directrion of creating a treatment that is ultimately aimed at helping the pelvic pain patient to create an inner environment in which the pelvic tissue irritability can heal. After all, the sore pelvic tissue is what is hurting and driving the other aspects of this self-feeding cycle.

Our program aims to break the self-feeding cycle by physically releasing sore pelvic muscles with our physical therapy self-treatment protocol, and then regularly immersing this tissue in a body whose nervous system is quiet and supportive of the recooperation and healing of the irritated tissue.

It's a three-part system: rehabilitation through release of pelvic floor related trigger points and stretching the myofascial tissue that has been constricted over the years, and *Extended Paradoxical Relaxation* (chapter 4), which regularly reduces anxiety and nervous system arousal. In this way, we aim to provide an environment for the tissue to ease tightening and allow the tissue irritability to heal.

Simple physical therapy, loosening the pelvic muscles and releasing pelvic trigger points, is only the first step.

> *Pelvic floor physical therapy alone, especially done*
> *by another and not regularly done by a patient*
> *carefully trained in pelvic floor physical therapy*
> *self-treatment, in our experience is inadequate by*
> *itself as a remedy for pelvic floor dysfunction.*

This critical understanding makes the difference between pelvic floor dysfunction resolving or not.

Most cases of chronic pelvic pain syndromes begin with a person's worry that regularly and sometimes unremittingly causes a reflex pelvic floor contraction.

The stressors that cause the pelvic floor to chronically tighten can be psychological or physical. What typically triggers symptoms of pelvic pain is the result of long-standing worry in which the pelvic floor is chronically tightened up. At times pelvic floor dysfunction can occur as the result of an intense physical or emotional trauma or a series of traumatic mental or physical stresses. Once set off, protective pelvic guarding/bracing aggravates and perpetuates already sore, painful pelvic floor muscles and a self-feeding cycle begins that takes on a life of its own.

The reason that chronic pain and dysfunction resist a simple mechanical fix is that the irritated pelvic muscles not only require release from contraction, but an ongoing quiet nervous system environment to allow the sore and irritated tissue to heal. The pelvic floor muscles are unique in that they are engaged much of the time and participate centrally in the normal daily functions of life, including urination, defecation, support and balance of the body, lifting, walking, sitting, and sexual activity among other activites. Without releasing the chronic contraction of the pelvic muscles and placing them in a *daily and extended healing environment,* the daily activities of life prevent the healing of the irritated pelvic muscle tissue.

A GUIDE TO THE PELVIC FLOOR

To understand pelvic pain, we need to be able to visualize the pelvic floor in relation to the rest of the body. Let's start with a very basic question many people with pelvic pain have—What and where is the pelvic floor?

If you think of the pelvis as a cereal bowl, the term *pelvic floor* refers to a group of muscles that can be thought of as the bottom of the cereal bowl. Tighten up the muscles you would use to interrupt urination, and you are tightening the muscles of your pelvic floor. When you generally tighten up your pelvic muscles you often also tighten the abdomen, the diaphragm, the inner thighs, and your sides.

In conventional stretching and strengthening practices, these pelvic muscles make up part of what are called the *core muscles.* They are required for posture, supporting the back to keep you straight and to keep you upright when your arms and legs move outward. If these muscles didn't exist to form a solid muscular girdle, you'd raise your arms or put your legs up and you'd fall over. It can be said that these muscles stabilize you during movement and hold the internal organs in place. Without them you couldn't walk, move, or lift anything. These muscles have to keep the center of the body stable for all different activities in life.

Generally speaking, the core muscles can't be seen in the way the biceps or calves can. You can tighten your pelvic muscles and most people would never notice it. They are hidden from view but play an essential role in life. Keeping them strong and healthy is the task of stretching and strengthening programs, like yoga and Pilates. These core muscles are places we sometimes tighten up when we're stressed. Having pelvic pain generally means being knotted up in these muscles. Resolving pelvic pain means dissolving a chronically tightened-up inner core.

THE THREE FUNCTIONS OF THE PELVIC FLOOR

Here we will briefly discuss the three functions of the pelvic floor: providing support, opening and closing the different orifices, and managing the symphony of sexual activity. Don't be overwhelmed reading this. We want to stay with the big picture of what the pelvic floor is, how pelvic pain can occur, and how to help it.

The pelvic muscles make it possible to control when you urinate and/or defecate. Think of the pelvic floor muscles as a hammock connected to the pelvic bones; three very important structures pass through this hammock. These structures are the vagina, whose muscles control childbirth and accommodate the penis during sexual intercourse; the urethra, which is the muscular tube connecting the bladder and providing passage of urine (and in men controlling the closing of the urethra and providing the passage of sperm during sexual activity through strong, rhythmic contractions); and the anorectal tube, which provides the passage of stool. The pelvic muscles allow for the voluntary control of both urination and defecation, and when you cough there is an involuntary contraction of the pelvic floor muscles to prevent urine or stool from leaking out as a result of the inner force in the core that would cause this kind of leakage.

Generally speaking, people who have no pelvic pain have pelvic muscles that tighten up and then relax. But for people who do have pelvic pain, whose way of expressing their anxiety is to tighten up the pelvis strongly and for a long time, or for people who have had some kind of injury and pain that has caused the pelvic muscles to reflexively tighten against the pain, the pelvic muscles don't relax well after contraction. They stay in a tightened state *or* ongoing spasm, and when the pelvic muscles don't relax, all kinds of weird symptoms occur.

Because the pelvic muscles are involved in so many complex and essential activities, chronically tightening up the pelvic muscles can create havoc in the interaction and communication between these muscles during vital activities. We all intuitively know this, although we may not know why. If anyone asked you to voluntarily tighten up for an hour the pelvic muscles that you would have to use to interrupt urination, no one would volunteer. Without knowing why, we intuitively know we don't want to go there. We don't want to tighten the pelvic muscles up for any extended period of time. People with pelvic pain often have chronically tightened up the pelvic muscles for years.

Let's return to the image of the pelvic floor as a cereal bowl made up of two parts: the bones of the pelvis, which are relatively rigid, and the muscles attached to the bones, which make up the bottom of the bowl. If the pelvis had only a bony structure and you put cereal and milk in it, they would all spill out. One of the important functions of the pelvic floor bowl is to hold up the inner organs.

Tension in the muscles in the bottom of the cereal bowl is connected to the legs, abdomen, sides, and back of the body. In other words, areas of pelvic restriction and places of trigger points referring into the pelvic muscles are found in the lower abdomen, buttocks, inner thighs, and places where nonpelvic muscles attach to the pelvic bones. Therefore, pelvic rehabilitation requires internal and external trigger point release, loosening of muscle constriction and stretching of both the inside and the outside of the pelvic floor, as well as many of the muscles immediately connected to the pelvis. This all being said, healing pelvic floor dysfunction is not accomplished simply by a mechanical release of tightened sore muscles without those muscles having the time and environment to stop being irritated and sore.

ADDRESSING PELVIC FLOOR PAIN AS A STATE OF CHRONICALLY IRRITATED PELVIC TISSUE

Problems can occur when the pelvic floor muscles are either weak or chronically tightened. Some practitioners confuse these two conditions and treat chronically tight pelvic muscles in the same way they would treat weak pelvic muscles.

Kegel exercises were originally meant to help women with weak pelvic muscles related to urinary incontinence by strengthening the muscles that connect the pubic bone to the sacrum, through which the urethra passes. Kegel exercises are in our view the very best and not harmful treatment for most cases of urinary incontinence. Chronically tightened pelvic muscles, however, do not benefit from being tightened by Kegel exercises. It's important to understand that weak pelvic muscles, and chronically tight and painful pelvic muscles are different problems requiring different solutions.

*Kegel exercises are generally not a good idea
if you have muscle-based pelvic pain.*

When someone has muscle-related pelvic pain, the muscles on the bottom of the pelvic cereal bowl are typically painful, tense, and shortened and contain knots of exquisite tenderness called trigger points, as well as areas of restriction and spasm. The pelvic tissue caught in the spasm does not have an opportunity to heal the way irritated tissue in other parts of the body can heal. These muscles can cause havoc with urination, defecation, orgasm, sexual arousal, and sitting. The goal of the *Wise-Anderson Protocol* is to restore these muscles to a loose, flexible, and comfortable state, allowing the irritated tissue to heal.

Normally, the pelvic floor muscles are dynamic, working and resting throughout the day. Even though they tighten, they have the ability to relax. The relaxed state allows for proper oxygenation, nutrition, blood flow, management of waste, and rejuvenation of tissue.

The pelvic floor muscles are not meant to be chronically contracted.

When muscles are chronically tensed, they tend to shorten, knot up, and eventually accommodate, so that the posture of a shortened state of the muscles feels uncomfortable but normal. People who have pelvic pain syndromes tend to focus tension in the pelvic muscles as a response to stress, anxiety, trauma, or pain.

When the pelvic muscles work too much, they can become painful. In all of the patients whom our protocol is able to help, stretching or pushing on at least some muscles of the pelvic floor or muscles outside the pelvic floor but related to it can cause pain or re-create symptoms. Our patients are often surprised when we tell them that these trigger points on a person without pelvic pain won't hurt when pressed. In fact, as someone's pelvic pain reduces or resolves, areas in and around the pelvis that once hurt when pressed will stop hurting.

The tendency to focus tension in the pelvic muscles is not an accident. Some have suggested that a person's inclination to focus tension in the pelvic muscles may begin with toilet training. The child is able to stop his parent's reaction to soiling by tightening his pelvic muscles. Over time, tightening the pelvis becomes a conditioned reaction to any situation in which anxiety arises. This idea of focusing tension in the pelvic muscles as a result of early toilet training is simply an idea, and we do not propose that it be taken as fact. It is, however, a compelling explanation of how pelvic tension may well begin early in life in some of our patients.

Research has shown, and it is our clinical experience as well, that people with chronic pelvic pain syndrome tend to have elevated pelvic floor tension even when resting. The pain and dysfunction get worse in the presence of stress. Many of our patients notice this relationship between stress and the severity in their symptoms. This observation leads to the heart of our understanding.

Sore, painful, chronically contracted pelvic muscle tissue is the very center of muscle-based pelvic pain. Even though soreness and chronic contraction are not detected by modern imaging techniques, they are as real as a broken bone.

Generally conventional medicine does not get excited about sore, shortened, contracted pelvic tissue. Conventional treatment has little to offer it. We believe that it is the very real physical basis of pelvic floor dysfunction and without resolving it pelvic pain continues. The purpose of the *Wise-Anderson Protocol* is to help in the healing of this sore pelvic tissue.

People who have chronic pelvic pain feel this soreness and irritation acutely. It sometimes feels like a burning, aching, tight, tearing, or very sore or raw area. When the doctor or physical therapist trained in trigger point release feels the inside of the rectum or vagina, or related external pelvic floor tissue, in patients with chronic pelvic pain syndromes, he or she often reports feeling areas of restriction, tension, and taut bands (trigger points) that, when touched, cause patients to jump with pain.

Some professionals who work inside the pelvic floor of people with pelvic pain describe the tissue as hard, restricted, tight, or rock-like. Areas within the pelvic floor that have been subjected to years of continual contraction need time to heal even when the muscles are no longer under tension. When physical therapy is done properly, and the pelvic floor is regularly rested, what feels like hardened tissue often becomes soft, supple, and pain-free. This is the goal of our treatment.

The inability of conventional diagnostic testing to detect any pathology does not mean that the debilitating condition of chronic pelvic pain does not exist. This inability is a limitation of the test technology.

Imagine tightening your fist as hard as you can for an hour. You will notice that there are places of lighter color in your hand that result from squeezing the blood out of the blood vessels. Your hand will feel uncomfortable, and you will feel relieved to stop the squeezing.

Now imagine you maintain this clenched fist for a day. Now imagine you maintain this fist for a week. Now imagine a month of tightening your fist constantly twenty-four hours a day. Now imagine doing it for a year. Now imagine doing it for several years. This is one way to understand the state of the pelvic floor in people with pelvic pain.

Imagine that, after several years, you stopped tightening your fist. Do you think the great discomfort and irritability of the tissues of your hand would immediately stop? Almost certainly not. It is not hard to imagine that you would want to rub your hand, massage it, and stretch out each finger to relieve it from the contracted state it had been in. Nor would it be hard to imagine that, even after you stopped tightening your fist, your fist would still be sore. It would take some time, some pampering, and most importantly, no chronic retightening of the fist before your hand felt normal again.

Many of our patients tend to be out of touch with what is going on in their pelvis. We offer a method to open communication with the pelvis to help bring about a healing of the sore and irritated pelvic tissues. We also aim to change patients' attitude toward their pelvis.

Resolving pelvic pain involves using physical and behavioral methods to restore the pelvic floor muscles to a relaxed and pain-free state while at the same time reducing the nervous system arousal that feeds pelvic floor tension and tissue irritability.

If chronic tension and nervous system arousal result in an irritation of the pelvic floor that gives rise to pain, then anything one does to reduce or eliminate the tension has the potential to help eliminate the pain. Practices that restore the contracted irritated tissues to a normal state of flexibility and relaxation have to be done repetitively.

It is the repetitive application of our methods that gives the pelvic muscles a chance to return to their normal state. We introduce the methods used to accomplish this, called *Extended Paradoxical Relaxation* and trigger point release. *Extended Paradoxical Relaxation,* discussed in depth in this book, trains the patient to break the habit of chronically tensing the pelvic muscles and chronically maintaining an aroused and anxious nervous system. Trigger point release makes it possible for the pelvic muscles to loosen. The physical therapy home self-treatment literally lengthens and softens the constricted pelvic tissue, allowing the sore tissue to heal.

> *The challenge in healing muscle-based pelvic pain*
> *is like the challenge of renovating a house while*
> *you are still living in it. It requires you to have*
> *patience and understanding of the healing process*
> *while still being engaged in normal functions of*
> *life that can irritate the already irritated tissue.*

There are important reasons why chronic pelvic pain syndromes are misunderstood and why healing is slow. One reason is that the pelvic muscles are almost always active in the service of the normal functions in life. The pelvic muscles need a rest from their chronic contraction, but two factors make this difficult. The first is that you can't simply rest the pelvic muscles for any extended period of time unless you are restfully sleeping or doing a method like *Extended Paradoxical Relaxation*. They are needed to allow you to stand up, to hold in urine and stool, to walk, to lift—to do the things that allow you to be able to function normally. It is a delicate juggling act to deal with both the need for rest and healing of this vital part of the body and the demand on the pelvic muscles to do the work required to function in life.

The second factor that operates against the healing of the pelvic floor is the tendency of many of our patients to live in a default, tensed-up state throughout the day, whether as a conditioned response to stress or as a natural biological response of protective guarding against pelvic pain. The tendency to tense the pelvis under stress is usually deeply ingrained, especially when it has been practiced many times without awareness. Modifying this habit so that contracting the pelvic muscles under stress is *not* the default mode is no small enterprise. Changing this habit is one of the main foci of the method of extended paradoxical relaxation.

For both these reasons, the process of healing takes time and much self-treatment, especially inside an active pelvic floor.

REASSURANCE AND EMOTIONAL SUPPORT

Harry Miller, M.D., from the department of urology at George Washington University, reported on his successful treatment of many men who had prostatitis through the use of a kind of stress management therapy. He gave patients simple and kindly advice not unlike that of a grandmother to her grandson. Miller's approach emphasized to his patients that there was a critical relationship between how they managed the stress in their life and their symptoms. In doing so, he helped most of his patients reduce their symptoms.

Miller's work focused on the person and not the prostate. He addressed the social and psychological context in which pelvic pain occurs. Similarly, the approach discussed in this book insists that prostatitis and related pelvic pain syndromes intimately involve a person's body and mind and are not limited to a sore part of the person's body independent of his mind and lifestyle.

A MULTIDISCIPLINARY TREATMENT TEAM

The *Wise-Anderson Protocol* is multidisciplinary and requires skills currently unavailable in any one conventional medical subspecialty. Its purpose is to teach patients how to heal themselves without having to rely on any further professional help. The team for the *Wise-Anderson Protocol* is composed of a urologist, a psychologist, and a physical therapist. It is unusual for these specialties to cooperate closely in the way that we do in the *Wise-Anderson Protocol,* and we consider it essential to our success. The physician does the initial diagnosis and makes sure that the condition is appropriate for our protocol. His or her work involves an examination of the patient, the administration of various medical tests, and interpretation of the results to rule out pathology. The physician or physical therapist examines and maps out the pelvic floor for trigger points and areas of restriction, then demonstrates intrapelvic trigger point release and trains patients to do this at home.

The psychologist's primary role is to train the patient in *Extended Paradoxical Relaxation* for the purpose of providing an inner environment for the sore pelvic tissue to heal. The psychologist on our team teaches a method to help the patient modify the difficult and often ingrained habit of catastrophic and negative thinking and default guarding that then becomes an integral part with the condition of pelvic pain and dysfunction. This method requires regular practice.

We believe that the best person to do our protocol is the patient him- or herself. A partner is *not* necessary for this protocol to be effective. The best physical therapy treatment for pelvic floor dysfunction is done by skilled patients who learn to do their own internal and external myofascial trigger point release. The physical therapist teaches the patient to self-administer the internal and external myofascial trigger point release and gives instructions for a home program of stretches, not unlike a home yoga program, except that these stretches are oriented toward the rehabilitation of the chronically tensed and irritated pelvic muscles. The relaxation protocol similarly must be done by the patient.

EFFECTIVE TREATMENT REQUIRES ADHERENCE TO THE COMPLETE PROGRAM

Our program requires at least two hours of self-treatment per day for many months. When self-treatment is successful in significantly reducing or stopping symptoms, some level of self-treatment is still required on a maintenance basis. Such a time commitment becomes easier as one becomes skilled in the method.

*Two hours plus of daily self-treatment
is recommended until symptoms abate,
while appearing daunting, it is necessary to
reverse the condition of years of chronically
contracted, sore pelvic muscles.*

REDUCING LIFE STRESS

Our treatment is most likely to help when you are willing to reduce the stress in your life.

John B., a thirty-eight-year-old small-business owner, came to see us at our clinic with pelvic pain and urinary dysfunction. Upon examining him, we determined that in fact he had no problems of an organic nature. He had trigger points inside his pelvic floor that when palpated exactly re-created his symptoms.

Under normal circumstances, John was someone we would be very optimistic about being able to help, but it became clear he was not. He owned a car repair facility where he employed forty-five people, and his business consumed his days from six in the morning until nine at night. His wife was unhappy because of his absence from their relationship. His children had behavioral and academic problems at school. He was also involved in a lawsuit with his brother-in-law, with whom he had owned a previous business. He was in the middle of a major renovation of his house that left both him and his wife sleeping on a mattress on the floor.

John had no time for himself, let alone the time to do physical therapy self-treatment and daily relaxation to relax his pelvic floor. Under these circumstances, the program we offered would have been ineffective because he would not have been able to do it properly in the face of the demands and stress calling for his attention. Only when John himself decided that his life would have to change would our treatment have a chance to help him resolve his pelvic pain.

One woman came to see us from overseas who had five children whom she was schooling at home. Aside from that daunting task, she held down a part-time job. Her husband offered her no assistance at home. The entire burden of raising and educating her children along with running the household fell on her shoulders. When she got away from her family and had time to do our protocol, her symptoms improved. In the normal course of her life, with no real time for herself, she floundered and her baseline level of symptoms remained.

This patient was very conflicted about taking any time for herself. Her idea was that she was selfish to take time for herself. Selfishness was to be shunned, so any time she took for herself felt almost like a sin. In these circumstances, her condition did not improve. This kind of attitude and lifestyle gives our protocol little chance of working. Daily self-treatment is the heart of our protocol. There is no way of shortchanging the time necessary for self-treatment if you want to benefit from what we have to offer.

*Those who are most successful in using our program
to reduce or resolve their symptoms are those who
have become experts in treating themselves.*

Patients who seem to get the best results find a way to commit themselves to earnest practice in our appraoch. Usually these patients have suffered for a long time and have seen numerous doctors and explored many avenues. They have done a variety of conventional treatments and have not been helped by these treatments. These patients often assume the attitude of "I will do whatever it takes to get better," and have no problem following the protocol.

*Like Home Depot, we give our patients the
message that "you can do it and we can help."*

Understanding that the treatment falls on your shoulders requires a shift in understanding about how healing occurs. Once we have instructed you in self-treatment, the responsibility for the treatment falls into your hands. The emphasis is that you can do it and are most likely to get results from our program when you take on that responsibility.

A PAINFUL PELVIS HAS TO BE COAXED
OUT OF ITS CONTRACTION

Just like a terrified kitten caught up a tree that has to be coaxed, soothed, and calmed down before it will cooperate, so too does the pelvis have to be coaxed into calming down. You can't reach it without appreciating its fear and its need for gentleness and consistency. If you approach it with anger, fear, resentment, impatience, or uncertainty, it will pick up your attitude and be more resistant to your help.

Strangely, relaxing a painfully contracted pelvis can create problems for the unconscious inner defenses. "How do I defend myself if I cannot guard my pelvis?" can be a major dilemma of the unconscious psychological defense system of the body. On the surface, this dilemma is irrational. Nevertheless, the unconscious defenses of the body are primitive, in our view often formed early in life, and not friendly to reason.

Typically, the pelvis has been tight for years, part of a default inner posture. This default inner posture remains in place despite all conventional and reasonable treatments. No drug has been able to fix this enormously distressing problem.

Healing muscle-related pelvic pain has its own rules. Antibiotics, sedatives, and muscle relaxants in the long term are of little use. Needles and knives often alienate the pelvis, creating more suffering. Even trigger point release that is not done in conjunction with relaxation as well as a change in attitude toward the symptoms tends to be at best short-lived.

The pelvis responds to kind, firm, patient coaxing. It responds to gentle persuasion. It responds to devotion and confidence in what you are doing. It responds to your being able to relax your fear and anger. It responds to your being able to regularly calm down your nervous system and free yourself from the grip of ongoing states of anxiety and storms of catastrophic thinking. It responds to your confidence in knowing where to press and loosen, both inside and outside your pelvis.

The painful pelvis can't be conned or coerced. The pelvis and the areas of the body around the pelvis must be lovingly and gently coaxed out of pain by supporting the healing of the sore, contracted pelvic tissue.

Chronic Pelvic Pain as a Functional Disorder

Muscle-based pelvic pain is not an irreversible pathology of structure, but a disturbance in function.

The closest that current medical paradigms come to understanding the nature of chronic pelvic pain syndromes, as we understand it, is using the concept of the functional somatic disorder. The concept of functional somatic disorder, or more simply, functional disorder, when applied to pelvic pain, can confuse a clear understanding.

When a researcher or doctor says that a condition is a functional disorder, he is usually saying that the source of the medical problem is not found in the physical structure but in the *functioning* of the structure.

For instance, in the functional disorder of irritable bowel syndrome, the tissue of the bowel is not pathological or sick but it behaves in a way that does not permit proper colonic processing, giving rise to bloating, motility dysfunction like diarrhea or constipation, pain and discomfort. The implication among many doctors is that functional disorders are in large part psychiatric.

We are proposing that the error in the concept of functional disorder regarding pelvic pain is that it paints a picture of the physical component of the problem as minor. A gastroenterologist will do a colonoscopy and, in the absence of ulceration, tumor, or infection, will report to the patient that there is nothing wrong with the colon. Perhaps he might note that the colon might appear contracted, but this is not seen to be remarkable. Similarly, the neurologist will look at a CAT scan (CT) of the brain and, in the absence of tumor, bleeding, or other gross pathology, will report that the findings were unremarkable.

Sore, contracted, trigger pointed pelvic tissue
does not show up on an MRI or CAT scan.
Nevertheless, in our view, healing this sore tissue
is the central issue in resolving pelvic floor pain.

What we are saying here is that the sore, irritated pelvic tissue is in fact a disturbance in structure, albeit not a life-threatening or irreversible one. While we believe that the physical findings of irritation, pain, increased muscle tension, trigger points, and spasticity are not indicative of gross pathology, they are in fact reversible. The centrality of resolving these symptoms is overlooked by most conventional approaches.

> *It is very common that our patients are told by their doctor that because all testing finds nothing remarkable, then there is nothing wrong with them, or that they should consider their problem mental and seek psychiatric counseling.*

Often, our patients feel dismissed by their doctors. Some patients have reported the doctor did not believe their complaints. This dismissal and invalidation of a patient's symptoms, on top of the huge distress of the symptoms, can create much suffering in the lives of those dealing with pelvic pain.

Simply, sore, irritated pelvic muscle tissue that appears to be the mildest kind of tissue disturbance, when in the grips of chronic pelvic tension, is the source of pelvic floor pain.

Is there something *physically* going on in the patient with pelvic pain that is not going on in the person without pelvic symptoms? The answer is unequivocally *yes*. But in the current medical model, soreness, trigger points, tissue hyperirritability, and chronic tension in response to this sore tissue are more or less considered minor events. Conventional medicine has little to help this tissue hyperirritability. The best medicine for this tissue hyperirritability is supporting the body's recuperative and healing capacity.

The point of this discussion is to make clear why our treatment intimately employs the skills of the psychologist, the physical therapist, and the physician. The *Wise-Anderson Protocol* must treat both the emotional/behavioral and physical components of pelvic pain. *Both are real and feed the self-feeding cycle. Furthermore, what is thought to be mental has real physical consequences,* as seen in the increased electrical activity in trigger points with increased anxiety that we see in the work of

RELATIONSHIP BETWEEN IRRITABLE BOWEL SYNDROME AND PELVIC PAIN

In our practice, we have noticed that there is a high incidence of irritable bowel syndrome in patients who also have pelvic pain. Given the proximity of the colon to the pelvis, it makes sense that both may well be the result of an aroused nervous system promotic chronic abdominal/pelvic tension and irritation of the chronically tightened tissue. While gastroenterology and urology make a distinction between the urogenital and gastrointestinal tract, the body has never heard of either specialty. Pelvic and gastrointestinal tightening often go hand in hand.

We will discuss in chapter 6 how the use of the *Wise-Anderson Protocol* with some slight variations has been helpful for some of our patients in reducing pain associated with irritable bowel syndrome and for a few patients in alleviating their distressing symptoms of esophageal reflux.

Richard Gevirtz and David Hubbard. People call up and ask whether we'll just do relaxation training in the absence of physical therapy or physical therapy in the absence of relaxation, and we tell them that we don't believe it is effective to break up our protocol this way.

THE CONCEPTS OF SYMPTOM THRESHOLD AND PELVIC PAIN

When first experiencing pelvic pain, one faces what seems to be a massive, pervasive discomfort and distress that feels incomprehensible and overwhelming. Patients usually feel helpless in the face of pelvic pain because they know little or nothing about what they can do about their condition. They don't understand what's happening to them and why and, most important, how to resolve it. Therefore, the concept of a threshold, and of proximity to the threshold, is often useful to help patients gain perspective on their progress.

We assess the effectiveness of our treatment by looking at the presence, intensity, and frequency of symptoms. Consider the following scheme. The symptom threshold is the point that your pelvic tension/tissue irritability reaches to cause painful irritation and reflex contraction in the pelvic floor. You can locate your proximity to the threshold, above which you are symptomatic and below which you are not. When patients are able to see their symptoms from the viewpoint of their proximity to the symptom threshold, they can sometimes better understand their situation.

Understanding the Often Baffling Symptoms of Pelvic Floor Dysfunction:
Proximity to the Symptom Threshold

#4   Chronically symptomatic
#3   Symptoms wax and wane when slightly above threshold

SYMPTOM THRESHOLD

#2   No symptoms when slightly below threshold; can
       become symptomatic at the slightest stress
#1   No symptoms

In the threshold schema, the person who is located in position #1 is well below the threshold of painful pelvic tissue irritation, displays no symptoms, and can tolerate a great amount of tension/nervous system arousal in the pelvic floor without becoming symptomatic. Even when this person's pelvic tension goes over the threshold, the pelvic tissue is not painfully irritated, and the pelvic floor muscles are flexible, so that they immediately drop below the threshold after the individual has stopped tensing. The person in this position has a normal, healthy pelvis.

The person situated in position #2 represents someone who likely will have pelvic pain but on an intermittent basis. It does not take great increases in pelvic tension/nervous system arousal level to irritate the pelvic tissue and go above the threshold where he or she will become symptomatic.

People with pelvic pain who are in position #2 are often bewildered at what brings on their symptoms. They conclude that little seemed to be associated with the onset or disappearance of symptoms and that the pain is random. Our explanation is that when someone is slightly below the threshold, what a nonevent would be for a normal person is often stressful enough to throw a #2 over the threshold and into symptoms.

At position #3 is the individual who has mild but persistent symptoms that wax and wane. This is the person who is "surfing" the threshold. Symptoms associated with #3, while seeming to be almost always present, occasionally drop below threshold, only to come back inexplicably. The person at position #3 usually experiences chronic but more or less tolerable pain/discomfort and dysfunction.

At position #4 is the individual who has chronic and intractable pelvic pain and/or dysfunction. He or she doesn't drop below the symptom threshold. When asked to describe the frequency and severity of symptoms, this person will report that the symptoms are always present, twenty-four hours a day, seven days a week, and that the symptoms strongly affect his or her life. Our treatment aims to lower baseline pelvic pain, the tension/neuromuscular irritability of individuals in positions #2, #3, and #4, to that of position #1.

In general, patients with pelvic floor dysfunction
pain have sore pelvic tissue when palpated—
people who do not have pelvic floor dysfunction
pain do not have sore pelvic tissue.

Most of the patients we see with chronic pelvic pain syndromes have what we have referred to earlier in this chapter as sore tightened tissue containing trigger points in their pelvis and related muscles. To reiterate, a trigger point is a taut band within a muscle that is painful either spontaneously or when touched and that creates pain at the site palpated or refers pain to a site remote from it.

Trigger points are exquisitely sensitive, and it is not uncommon for the patient to jump when the trigger point is pressed. We determine the presence of a trigger point through a digital/rectal or digital/vaginal examination for internal trigger points. The doctor inserts a finger inside the rectum or vagina and presses on the muscles to assess the tissue and to find trigger points. External trigger points are evaluated using the methodology described by Janet Travell and David Simons in *Myofascial Pain and Dysfunction: The Trigger Point Manual.*

A 1994 study sheds much light on the relationship between trigger points and stress. Walter McNulty, Richard Gevirtz, David Hubbard, and Gregory Berkoff inserted a needle electrode directly into a trigger point and monitored its electrical activity with a machine called an electromyograph. It appears that the higher the electrical activity in a trigger point, the higher the level of pain.

Patients were given the stressful task of doing mental arithmetic. The scientists wanted to determine what the effects of stress were on the trigger points being monitored and the differences, if any, between the responses of the trigger points and the responses of the adjacent nonsensitive tissue without trigger points. Results indicated that the electrical activity of the trigger points increased during this stressful activity while the adjacent, non–trigger point tissue remained essentially electrically unresponsive.

This kind of experiment has been replicated hundreds of times. These findings are remarkable. They suggest that in some way the nervous system that is connected to the stress of emotional activity and arousal is selectively connected to trigger points and not to non–trigger point tissue. The findings make clear why patients with pelvic pain and dysfunction routinely report that their symptoms are aggravated by stress.

Plato taught that we need to be kind to each other because each of us is engaged in a mighty, yet unseen, struggle in our lives. Compassion for the most difficult of people comes from understanding their struggle. Like letting go of anger and fear toward difficult people, letting go of fear and anxiety toward a painful rectum and genitals is simply an expression of your understanding and compassion for your own struggle.

Developing patience and compassion
toward flare-ups can help reduce their
pain, symptoms, and duration.

Discovering compassion toward oneself and one's body is part of our protocol. As patients understand the language of the pelvic floor and their struggle with their habit of chronically tightening it, their attitude can change from fear to compassion and understanding.

The self-feeding cycle of tissue soreness–
anxiety–pain–reflex–protective
guarding: the heart of the problem.

Chronic pelvic pain has been resistant to effective treatment because of what we call the *tissue soreness–anxiety–pain–protective guarding cycle*. This is a self-feeding cycle of chronic reflex pelvic tension causing the formation of painful irritation in muscles in the pelvic floor. Together with the physical effects of anxiety in the trigger points of the contracted, irritated tissue, a self-feeding cycle forms that makes it appear that the condition has a life of its own.

THE SELF-FEEDING CYCLE OF PELVIC PAIN

Tissue Soreness/Anxiety/Pain/Protective Guarding Cycle

ANXIETY
chronic
anxiety/worry

PELVIC TENSION
chronic tension of the
pelvic floor muscles

DAILY ACTIVITIES
TRIGGER SYMPTOMS
activities of daily life block
pelvic tissue healing and
promote more pain

PELVIC TISSUE
SORENESS
over time painful/non-
pathological pelvic muscle
soreness develops

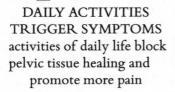
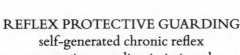

REFLEX PROTECTIVE GUARDING
self-generated chronic reflex
protective guarding in irritated
pelvic muscles

Once the pelvis becomes sore and painful and the normal functions are disturbed in some way, that sore and painful pelvis becomes hypersensitive to anxiety. Anxiety results in the tightening of the muscles in preparation for fight, flight, or freeze. This tightening of the pelvic floor and surrounding musculature tends to be reflexive and usually happens outside of a person's awareness.

Some level of anxiety is what almost all patients with chronic pelvic pain syndromes live with day in and day out. Anxiety can regularly exacerbate the condition fed by the patient's catastrophic thinking, the isolation of sharing one's feelings with very few, and a medical establishment that can't help.

> *Pelvic pain is hugely affected and perpetuated by anxiety. This is why the placebo effect reduces the anxiety that helps fuel the condition.*

This is also why many people have a reduction in symptoms after they read this book. Finally something makes sense about what is going on and offers some intuitively viable answer.

PELVIC PAIN AND THE RESPONSE OF "PULLING THE TAIL BETWEEN THE LEGS"

In 2009, after the printing of the fifth edition of our book, an insight occurred to us about pelvic pain. This insight helps clarify the pervasiveness of muscle-related pelvic pain and its biological basis. It is common knowledge that a dog will pull his tail between his legs when he is fearful. Other emotions have been attributed to this tail-pulled-between-the-legs behavior, including shame, submission, dread, defeat, and shyness. For the present discussion, we propose here that the common denominator running through the various emotions associated with the tail-pulled-between-the-legs behavior is fear.

In the typology of Walter Cannon, the Harvard physiologist of the early twentieth century who introduced the phrase *fight, flight, freeze* to describe the varieties of survival behavior in mammals, a tail pulled between the legs is an expression of the survival behavior that he termed *freeze*. This *freeze* behavior expresses the organism's attempt to self-protectively hold fast while waiting for danger to pass. The behavior of a waving tail has been associated among animal watchers with the emotions of excitement or aggression, contrasting sharply to the tail-pulled-between-the-legs behavior. Most cat and dog owners, for example, intuitively read their animals' emotional states, in large part, by what the tail is doing.

In humans, the tailbone is commonly understood to be what remains of the tail inherited from our humanoid ancestors. This tailbone (coccyx) is sometimes called the vestigial tail. In humans, the coccygeal, iliococcygeal, and pubococcygeal muscles of the pelvic basin are attached to the coccyx or tailbone and are responsible for its movement, in conjunction with other pelvic floor muscles.

The phrase "tail between the legs" exists in the vernacular of many languages to describe behaviors of fear, shame, submission, cowardice, or defeat. For example, in French, the term *la queue entre les jambes* is commonly used and is identical in meaning to "tail between the legs." In modern Greek, the transliterated phrase *Autos einai san to skylo pou vazi tin oura mes ta skelia tou* translates as "He is like the dog who puts his tail deep down below." Greeks often use this phrase to describe someone who is fearful, anxious, nervous, ashamed, or beaten down by life. Interestingly as well, the phrase is often used to describe someone who can't make a decision, who is "frozen" by choices before him and obsesses over which decision to make.

> *Muscle-based pelvic pain can be thought*
> *of as a condition resulting from pelvic floor*
> *irritation caused by chronically "pulling*
> *the tail" in between one's legs.*

The phenomenon of pulling the tail between the legs requires that specific pelvic floor muscles, particularly involving the coccygeal muscles, participate in this muscular event. In this act of muscle contraction, this set of pelvic muscles contracts, causing the tail (tailbone) to pull in. We offer the insight here that in terms of evolution the tail pulled between the legs is an active behavior associated with the experience of fear and that its likely aim is to protect the anorectal area and genitals of the organism. This behavior also signals to a predator or competitor that the animal offers no threat.

Sitting Pain and the Reflex of Pulling the Tail Between the Legs

To our knowledge, in the scientific discussion of pelvic pain, there has been no discussion of what we believe to be the intimate relationship between tail-pulled-between-the-legs behavior, anxiety, and pelvic pain. Here we introduce this idea and the therapeutic implications of this surprisingly clinically important relationship.

The muscles required to "pull in the tail"
are typically painful or sore in those with
discomfort related to sitting down.

From the beginning of our research, we have known that pelvic pain was related to chronic self-protective muscle tension that formed a self-feeding cycle of tension-anxiety-pain and protective guarding.

The biological instinct for animals to pull the tail between the legs exemplifies why pelvic pain, to one degree or another, exists in human beings regardless of race, gender, or country of origin. Muscle-based pelvic pain may come from a universal, biologically based behavior that appears to be hard-wired in vertebrates.

The insight that pelvic pain is related to tail-pulled-between-the-legs behavior has both theoretical and practical applications. The practical application more clearly identifies what we believe is the therapeutic strategy necessary to treat posterior symptoms like sitting pain, coccygeal pain, and post–bowel movement pain in particular, along with associated pelvic pain and dysfunction in general.

The Muscles That "Pull the Tail Between the Legs" Are the Muscles Most Associated with Pelvic Pain

Upon examination, the muscles involved in the tail-pulled-between-the-legs behavior are among the most common trigger-pointed, shortened, irritated, and painful muscles in patients with pelvic pain. In the data we have collected from patients who have visited us for treatment of their pelvic pain, we have very often been able to re-create pain associated with sitting coccygeal pain and post–bowel movement pain by palpating the iliococcygeus, pubococcygeus, puborectalis, sphincter ani, gluteus maximus, and piriformis muscles.

It is also important to say that physical trauma or injury to the pelvis can trigger this protective tail-pulled-between-the-legs behavior. In other words, the tail-pulled-between-the-legs behavior can occur outside states of chronic anxiety or fear. The tail-pulled-between-the-legs phenomenon is essentially invisible to our fellow humans because we do not have a visible tail to inform each other of our states of fear and anxiety. Because muscle-related pelvic pain likely has its origins in this biological instinct, it makes sense that this disorder consists of various spastic or chronically contracted muscles that tighten the entire pelvic floor and are fed by tissue irritation, tension, anxiety, pain, and protective guarding. Once set in motion, this syndrome takes on a life of its own and forms a self-feeding cycle, even when the fearful event or trauma has passed.

Sitting pain is one of the last symptoms to resolve when our approach is successful in treating muscle-based pelvic pain.

The amelioration of sitting pain requires not only the rehabilitation of the taut, chronically tensed irritated muscles that result from a biological impulse to pull the tail between the legs in states of fear but also a lowering of the default level of nervous system arousal whose absence keeps the tail chronically pulled in. Lowering the default level of nervous system arousal requires ongoing practice in reversing the thinking process representing the world as a dangerous place in which we must remain protectively guarded. *Extended Paradoxical Relaxation* provides a regular time during the day when you can release your protective guarding, free yourself from fear, and inwardly rest. In the moments of being free from anxiety, the biological reflex to keep the tail pulled in is interrupted and the pelvic floor can get accustomed to being relaxed.

COGNITIVE THERAPY

If we look at the slang related to the anal sphincter, we typically will hear someone on the street referring to someone as a "tight-ass" or being "anal." Using this term to refer to someone tends to mean that they are perfectionistic, withholding, cheap, or obsessed with detail. It relates the tightness of the anal canal to such psychological and characterological traits. The "tight-ass" is just a certain kind of person. These terms imply that your character (and the state of your pelvis) is like the color of your eyes or the enduring characteristics of a personality. It is remarkable to notice how these terms have become part of the vernacular, when they first originated in obscure psychoanalytic theory. What Freud referred to as "anal" was derived from a psychological fixation associated with the anal phase of development.

It is a new paradigm to think you can voluntarily relax your habitually tight core, which includes the anorectal area. When you call someone a "tight-ass," the implication is that such a person is characteristically in a chronic state—someone who is "tight-assed" or "anal" is considered a kind of person whose habitual tendency is to be perfectionistic, compulsive, or picayune and cannot be reformed. Our protocol is based on the understanding that concerted voluntary efforts to behaviorally change the default tone of the anal sphincter and other muscles of the pelvic floor, can change one that is tight and chronically contracted to one that is relaxed and at ease.

Unfortunately, behavioral treatment for anal fissures to reduce the high muscle tone of the anal sphincter is not generally a focus of colorectal surgeons who are consulted for this problem. If you seek treatment from a colorectal surgeon, you may well end up having surgery. This conventional approach of surgery does not take into consideration the fact that someone with a tight anal sphincter can learn to voluntarily loosen it and thereby restore normal blood flow with proper physical therapy and behavioral instruction.

It is possible for many to relax a chronically contracted anal sphincter to a normal tone without drugs or surgery.

Over a lifetime, we believe that teaching people to calm down their insides under their own volition is by far the most cost-effective method of dealing with pelvic pain that exists, despite the fact that initially training people to do this has its costs. In our view, the psychophysical treatment of the *Wise-Anderson Protocol* represents the best framework within which someone can modify a chronically contracted core.

A Gentle Approach to Break the Sore Tissue–Anxiety–Pain–Protective Guarding Cycle

The *Wise-Anderson Protocol* intervenes in all aspects of the self-feeding cycle of tissue soreness–anxiety–reflex protective guarding. *Extended Paradoxical Relaxation* lowers pelvic tension and anxiety by lowering autonomic nervous system arousal and importantly by providing a regular healing chamber for the sore pelvic tissue to heal. *Trigger Point Release* and certain myofascial release methods, including what we describe as *skin rolling* and *pelvic floor yoga,* deactivates trigger point pain, lengthens chronically contracted muscles, all to enable a hospitable environment for the healing of the chronically sore and irritated pelvic tissue.

When someone is caught in the grip of the self-feeding cycle of tissue soreness–anxiety–pain and reflex protective guarding, we are certain of the necessity of doing internal and external trigger point release gradually and gently. While a flare-up of symptoms when doing internal trigger point release is common, it is generally to be avoided. We generally do not agree about doing trigger point release that causes regular flare-ups of symptoms. If the patient cannot tolerate any pressure inside the rectum or vagina, we begin the physical part of our treatment by simply inserting a finger with no pressure anywhere. If they cannot tolerate the insertion of the finger, we hold the finger gently, touching the opening of the rectum or vagina without moving at all. In backing up and reducing the intensity of the treatment to a tolerable level, we find a baseline from which to begin.

John J., a patient from Minneapolis, could not tolerate any pressure inside his pelvic floor. When we instructed his wife in the *Trigger Point Release*, we told her to simply insert her finger inside his rectum and not press anywhere. She did this on a daily basis for a week, and with our instruction, she began slightly pressing on a trigger point. Gradually, as her husband could tolerate more, she increased the pressure. After a few months, he was able to tolerate the pressure that we are usually able to exert at the beginning of treatment with most other patients. Similarly, John J. was not able to lie down and do the first lesson in the relaxation training for more than three minutes. We instructed him to do *Paradoxical Relaxation* for two minutes each day, which he did for a week or so. Following this, we asked him to increase the relaxation time gradually until he reported actually relaxing for over a period of half an hour.

HOW OUR TREATMENT WORKS

Daily Treatment

> *Our intention is to help our patients give
> their sore and irritated pelvic muscles and
> structures an opportunity to heal.*

Our method for doing this is "low tech" and not "high tech." We ask our patients to do two-plus hours of self-treatment daily. This typically goes on for many months and sometimes a few years. Furthermore, patients are instructed to practice momentarily releasing the habitual tension in the pelvic floor many times a day by doing *Moment-to-Moment Paradoxical Relaxation*. This is not a small matter. The pelvic muscles rebel against being bullied or beaten up by aggressive and insensititive levels of pressure that regularly cause flare-ups. We discuss this in the "pressure principle" related to how much pressure should be used in doing internal trigger point release.

While during the first number of sessions of *Trigger Point Release* inside the pelvic floor, there can be a flare-up of symptoms, often lasting between a few hours to several days or longer, we have come to instruct our patients to use pressure that causes little or no flare-up even if it feels like the pressure is hardly any pressure at all.

The full effectiveness of our protocol for an individual cannot be known until after it is actually done and the effects are evaluated. It does not help everybody. We always evaluate the appropriateness of our treatment according to a patient's symptoms and recommend it after a urologic evaluation when it is clear that there is no gross pathology and when, according to our experience, the patient is likely to benefit. In other words, even if you fit our criteria as an appropriate candidate and we believe you are likely to significantly benefit from our protocol, there is no way of determining the exact level of effectiveness of our treatment for you until you do it earnestly and observe the results.

Our approach does not use drugs, surgery, or invasive procedures. In fact, our goal is to help patients off all drugs. Every patient is examined with a traditional urologic workup, and disorders of infection, obstruction, or neurological abnormality are treated appropriately.

The Purpose of Our Protocol Is to Help Our Patients Become Independent of Doctors and Health Professionals

We teach our patients how to help themselves. Our purpose is to make our patients free of dependency on professionals. A partner is not necessary for the success of our protocol. If the patient would like the partner to help, we can help train the partner.

Our protocol can help a select group of patients with muscle-based pelvic pain significantly reduce their symptoms or become essentially symptom-free.

> *The most important benefit that our protocol*
> *offers is the real possibility of helping selected*
> *individuals with muscle-related pelvic*
> *pain significantly reduce their symptoms*
> *or essentially become symptom-free.*

Because pelvic pain tends to recur under periods of stress, our protocol gives the patients the tools that empower them to help resolve their own symptoms. This is of great value. Furthermore, as symptoms reduce, a continued improvement in symptoms tends to be ongoing for many patients if they sincerely comply with the protocol and competently manage their response to stress.

Our Values and Assumptions
1. Above all, do no harm.
2. Help our patients by putting them beyond the need for our help.
3. Regularly being able to reduce or stop the pain and symptoms of pelvic pain is the best therapy for doubt and catastrophic thinking.
4. Eagerness and earnestness make the possibility of our protocol helping most likely.
5. Action is the proof of earnestness.
6. Faith and belief are not necessary in doing our protocol—daily practice of our protocol is essential.
7. It is what you do that counts. The only way to know the extent to which our protocol can help you is by doing it and seeing the results.
8. Pelvic pain didn't start overnight and it doesn't go away overnight.

9. Resolving muscle-related pelvic pain ultimately is an inside job.

10. The aspiration to dissipate fear, discomfort, and tension by learning to relax with it makes our protocol most likely to work.

CHAPTER 3

THE *WISE-ANDERSON PROTOCOL*, PART 1: *TRIGGER POINT RELEASE*

Pelvic floor–related trigger point release is a manual self-treatment technique of deactivating pain-referring trigger points and stretching, loosening, and lengthening the contracted tissue inside and outside the pelvic floor, thereby enabling it to relax. The technique focuses on trigger points and areas of spasm and constriction related to pelvic pain. In the *Wise-Anderson Protocol,* patients are taught to self-administer trigger point release inside and outside the pelvic floor. That said, the detailed information on trigger point release techniques in this chapter should not be used as a substitute for proper in-person physical therapy training. We do not recommend patients treat themselves internally. Competent performance of our physical therapy protocol is not mastered by reading a description of it but comes from in-person instruction and experience in successfully working with trigger point release particularly inside the pelvic floor.

> *Skill at doing pelvic floor physical therapy self-treatment, especially internally, comes with clear instruction and regular practice of self-treatment.*

Trigger Point Release aims to help our patients free the muscles in and around their pelvis of active trigger points and to restore the muscles of the pelvic floor to a flexible, lengthened, soft, and supple state. This is done by teaching patients a specialized type of internal and external therapy that deactivates painful trigger points and rehabilitates the soft tissue of the pelvic floor. In this aspect of treatment, a patient is in direct physical contact with the physical sites of the pain and constriction. We teach patients to do trigger point release on themselves with their finger, our FDA-approved Internal Trigger Point Wand, our Trigger Point Genie, and other methods.

GETTING OFF DRUGS

One of the goals of the *Wise-Anderson Protocol* is to help our patients get off all drugs. This often is not possible at the beginning of treatment. Many patients have been given antibiotics, alpha blockers, muscle relaxants, and painkillers. Not infrequently, patients have grown reliant on pain-reducing analgesics in order to cope with their symptoms.

While it is sometimes possible for patients to wean themselves off these medications before treatment, this is in no way essential.

We now suggest patients remain on their medications and slowly wean off them, under physician supervision, once their self-treatment begins to reduce their pain.

In general, we do not support the use of narcotic pain medicines because they tend to lower a person's pain threshold and often lead to habituation or addiction. We recognize that some individuals' pelvic pain is so great and debilitating that narcotic medication has been the only relief, or partial relief, that they have had. There are patients whom we have helped who began treatment while taking narcotic medications and have been able to wean themselves off these medications during the course of their self-treatment.

RE-CREATING SYMPTOMS THROUGH TRIGGER POINT PALPATION

We have had our best results when we have been able to find trigger points internally and/or externally, or have been able to stretch contracted or spastic muscles that tend to re-create some aspect of a patient's symptoms. Determining whether someone has trigger points requires the evaluation of someone experienced in trigger point release and physical therapy for pelvic pain. Later in this chapter, we describe and show illustrations of the most common trigger points related to pelvic pain.

Some readers have written us to ask if an unremarkable biofeedback reading rules them out for our protocol. A pelvic floor biofeedback reading is an unreliable criterion for determining the appropriateness of our protocol. In other words, a rectal or vaginal biofeedback sensor that indicates a normal amount of tension on any particular machine is not a reason to rule out the appropriateness of our protocol. Pelvic floor electromyographic evaluation of the anal sphincter or the opening of the vagina is one of those medical tests in which a positive finding may be significant and point toward the proper therapy, whereas a negative result does not prove anything.

MAKING A PAIN-FREE STATE THE NORMAL STATE

No one with pelvic pain and dysfunction says that his or her symptoms feel comfortable or normal. However, over time, your body may have adapted to your pain and dysfunction as a peculiar kind of normal state. In other words, your pelvic pain and dysfunction at a certain level may become an uncomfortable "home" and a place that feels stable.

It is often the case that patients will experience significant relief from symptoms after both *Extended Paradoxical Relaxation* and *Trigger Point Release*. This relief is often brief, with symptoms reemerging after hours or days. In our view, the "normal" setting was shifted from one of pain to one of less or no pain. This setting needs to be reestablished as "normal" by repeating treatment over and over again. *One purpose of the* Wise-Anderson Protocol *is to retrain the nerves, muscles, and blood vessels so that freedom from pain and dysfunction feels like home as chronically irritated pelvic tissue heals.*

DEFINING *TRIGGER POINT RELEASE* AND *MYOFASCIAL RELEASE*

Our patients are often confused about the difference between trigger point release and myofascial release. The typical reference to myofascial/trigger point release makes it appear that they are one method when actually they are two different methods. While we clearly use myofascial release methods, *we believe that they are not by themselves an effective treatment for pelvic pain.* We wish to be clear that in the *Wise-Anderson Protocol* the strong emphasis is on trigger point release, though we do use myofascial release methods as well.

Trigger point release is a method of identifying and releasing knots or taut bands in muscles that often refer pain to a site remote from the actual trigger point. *Myofascial release* is a name given to stretching the fascia, or connective tissue around muscles, that over time has tightened up and restricted the muscles that it surrounds.

Our treatment has evolved over (at the time of this printing) the past twenty-four years, and our experience has taught us that patients do best with our protocol when they learn to use it themselves. Therefore our treatment involves teaching patients how to regularly interrupt the self-feeding cycle of tension, anxiety, and pain, which is the heart of the pelvic pain syndromes we treat, and how to keep the muscles in the pelvis loose, unrestricted, and pain-free. The resolution of pelvic pain is an inside job.

DEACTIVATING TRIGGER POINTS AND REHABILITATING THE CHRONICALLY IRRITATED AND KNOTTED-UP PELVIC FLOOR

It may seem like a challenge for most people to gently reach inside the pelvic floor with a gloved, lubricated finger or wand, rectally or vaginally, in order to release pelvic pain–related trigger points, spasm, and areas of restriction. In fact, it is relatively easy to do once one's initial reluctance and awkwardness are overcome. Indeed, while doing internal trigger point release may sound strange, people do far more invasive kinds of self-treatment, like routinely injecting themselves with insulin or catheterizing themselves in order to urinate. Trigger point release, especially at the beginning of therapy, in the scheme of things, is relatively easily done and unremarkable but does require some level of instruction from an experienced practitioner.

We have heard from many people with pelvic pain who have bought some kind of sex toy that they inserted internally for the purpose of doing *Trigger Point Release*. These toys are typically designed for sexual stimulation, are not approved by the FDA, and we don't recommend them for this purpose.

WE GENERALLY DO NOT RECOMMEND TRIGGER POINT INJECTIONS

Some doctors use needles inside the pelvic floor to do *Trigger Point Release*. We do not think this is a good idea for a number of reasons. First of all, it is difficult to identify a trigger point and then accurately insert a needle into it inside the pelvic floor. Second, the area cannot be made sterile, and for reasons related to hygiene and infection there is some risk involved. We have had patients who had severe reactions to needles being inserted inside the pelvic floor, from the inadvertent piercing of a blood vessel that filled the abdomen with blood to painful flare-ups that lasted months after a nerve was probably nicked. Furthermore, the use of needles promotes the idea that the pelvic floor cannot be helped by oneself but only by a professional. This is an idea we do not support.

In general, we think that a self-treatment tool inserted into the pelvic floor is useful only where one cannot reach with one's own finger. Toward this end, we have developed the only FDA-approved self-treatment Internal Trigger Point Wand to deactivate internal trigger points that are difficult for a patient to deactivate manually.

We think that the use of a finger, carefully supervised, is superior to any instrument because when you use your finger you are the therapist and the patient at the same time and your feedback to yourself is immediate. In other words, you can feel the area that you are working on, as well as feel and adjust the level of pressure you are exerting.

Finally, with regard to teaching patients to do internal trigger point release, we believe that a professional needs to have the experience of competently doing an internal self-treatment on him- or herself before teaching a patient to do so.

THE NECESSITY FOR
REPETITIVE TREATMENT

Trigger Point Release needs to be done very gradually and repetitively so that offending trigger points become quiet and the pelvic muscles remain relaxed for extended periods of time to facilitate healing of the irritated pelvic tissue.

The actual number of self-treatment sessions varies. We encourage patients to use internal trigger point release and myofascial release after coming to our clinic between two to four times per week. These methods have to be used repetitively in order to override the tendency of the pelvic floor to remain irritated and contracted when it has been so for a prolonged period of time.

In doing *Trigger Point Release,* we are saying to the tissue:

We know you are distressed, we know you are hurting, we know you are irritated and contracted. We are going to press on painful trigger points in you to release them. We are going to stretch you to give you room to breathe, to be nourished, and to rest. At first it will probably hurt because you are used to being tense and contracted, so any stretching that we do to you will probably feel uncomfortable and unknown. You are used to being uncomfortable and so any sense of comfort, while feeling good, may not feel like "home" to you. We remind you over and over again that it is okay to lengthen and soften and relax. We are going to stretch you regularly so that the lengthened state becomes normal for you. As we do this, the gentle stretching may be both uncomfortable and paradoxically may also feel good. It may sometimes feel like the discomfort of what is being done to you during a session "hurts so good." We do this as your friend and want the best for you. We know that when you learn that it is okay to be out of pain, you will want to stay out of pain. We want you to feel safe. Let's work together.

WHAT TO EXPECT FROM
TRIGGER POINT RELEASE

In our own practice on the first day of our six-day immersion clinic, our physical therapist will privately examine patients externally, and feel and evaluate all of the muscles that relate to the pelvic floor. Our physical therapist determines whether there are trigger points or constriction in them. He will palpate trigger points to see if they refer pain into the areas where you are symptomatic.

The external examination first assesses muscles of the trunk and lower abdomen, looking for acute trigger points that may refer symptoms to the pelvic region.

Both the examination and the treatment of the inside of the pelvic floor. In the male patient this is done privately while the man is lying in the prone position (on his stomach) with pillows under his pelvis. This position is an innovation of Tim Sawyer. Occasionally the man will be examined and treated in the lithotomy position (on the back with knees bent and open). Women can be examined either prone, on their side, or on their back, depending on the area of the pelvic floor that needs to be reached.

When evaluating and mapping the trigger points, our physical therapist reaches inside of the pelvis either vaginally or rectally with a gloved finger, liberally lubricated to avoid chafing or irritating the pelvic tissue. In rectal-related treatment, we begin by entering the rectum and examining the sphincter ani (the rings of muscle at the opening of the rectum), then moving to the coccygeus muscle, and then moving to the back, middle, and front of the levator ani muscles. The therapist carefully checks the obturator internus muscle because of its relationship to the pudendal nerve, which runs through the pelvis and posterior ligaments.

The therapist may examine the left side of the body using the right hand, and the right side of the body using the left hand. Using the finger as the instrument of treatment requires the therapist to be in a certain position to gain maximum strength in palpating and stretching the trigger points. Using the hand that is opposite the side of the patient's pelvic floor (right hand to the left pelvic floor, and left hand to the right pelvic floor) affords maximum leverage and extension inside.

In digital rectal examination of male patients, the therapist works with the trigger points that are often found in the insertions of the muscles into the pelvis around the prostate. We do not do prostate massage or work on the prostate gland. As the therapist assesses and works with the trigger points on the edge of the prostate, we move into the anterior, then middle, then posterior levator ani muscles, and then the piriformis and coccygeus muscles. In a ninety-degree position (with the finger perpendicular), the therapist moves to the side wall of the pelvis to assess the obturator muscles.

An evaluation generally starts outside the pelvis, including the lower abdominal and oblique muscles with the trigger points found, as it helps prepare the patient for internal work. The treatment of the external muscles consists of trigger point release and stretching of soft tissue, followed by heat and instructions for the home stretching program. The therapist examines and treats the following muscles: abdominals, psoas, quadratus lumborum, gluteals, piriformis, adductors, pectineus, and paraspinals. The therapist works on these muscles with the patient lying in different postures to facilitate lengthening of the tissue and to deactivate trigger points during this phase of treatment. In our clinic, the focus of our sessions with patients, again, is training each patient in self-treatment.

In our own clinical examinations, we use a three-point system to identify the levels of pain and tenderness of the trigger points (0 = no pain, 1+ = mild pain, 2+ = moderate pain, 3 = severe pain). When trigger points are pressed, very often the pressure will prompt someone to jump. This is called "the jump sign" and is one of the tests verifying the existence of a trigger point. When there is a jump response, or a very tender area, we indicate that by using the designation 3+.

TECHNIQUES USED INSIDE THE PELVIC FLOOR

We use several techniques. The most common is called the *pressure/release technique*. It has also been called the technique of *ischemic compression*. You will understand this method if you apply pressure to the back of your left hand with your right index finger. You will notice that when you press on the back of your hand and then release it, a little white spot is temporarily created where the blood was momentarily pushed out by the finger pressure. This is what we do inside the pelvic floor.

We feel for the typical "taut band," characteristic of the trigger point, and apply pressure to it to help release it. We hold this pressure for approximately fifteen to ninety seconds, while always staying in communication with our patient about his or her level of discomfort. Pressing on trigger points like this, especially at first, can be quite uncomfortable. The tolerance patients have for pressure release of trigger points is improved to the extent to which they feel they can control the duration and intensity of the pressure. We proceed systematically throughout the pelvic floor, applying this pressure release technique.

It is important to relax while doing trigger point release so that the tissue is not tightening up against the pressure that aims to lengthen and release it.

We sometimes use another technique, developed by George Thiele in the 1940s, though we regard Thiele massage alone as an inadequate treatment technique. His method involves a sweeping motion, stroking the length of the muscle. We sometimes stroke or apply pressure to a trigger point until we feel it lengthen and soften. At that point we ask the patient to tighten the muscle while we press against it. Then we ask the patient to relax and let go of the tightening. This method helps lengthen and soften certain rigid pelvic muscles.

After a patient is instructed in trigger point release with the finger and with our Internal Trigger Point Wand, the discomfort of both the external and internal trigger points tends to diminish, and we are left with certain remaining and often stubborn, sore trigger points. We ask patients, when it is possible for them, to take hot baths before a self-treatment session as a way of helping loosen muscles that are tight and constricted. We often suggest a warm compress to patients or ask them to take a warm bath after treatment as well.

We tell patients that they may have flare-ups throughout treatment. This is a very important communication, because if the patient's expectation is that there will be a steady and unflagging improvement in symptoms, the flare-up after treatment can feel like a defeat and an invalidation.

In the first evaluation, a flare-up of symptoms can be seen positively because it tends to corroborate our diagnosis and it tells us that we are in the right place. As self-treatment and physical therapy continue, pain and discomfort associated with it tend to diminish, although very uncomfortable flare-ups that hearken back to the level of the original symptoms do happen from time to time and are not a bad thing. We ask our patients to be exceedingly gentle especially in performing internal trigger point release.

There is no formula determining exactly the minimum or maximum number of treatments required to achieve success with the physical therapy method used in the *Wise-Anderson Protocol*. Some patients respond immediately and require only minimal rehabilitation of the internal and external pelvic-related musculature coordinated with good *Extended Paradoxical Relaxation* practice. Some patients need extensive treatments because of a tendency to return to a baseline tension level. We encourage patients to do self-treatment regularly until painful and constricted tissue softens and stops being painful when stretched or pressed.

Windows of symptom abatement typically occur, though not always, soon after treatment begins. The reliable ongoing reduction or absence of symptoms usually takes much time and great patience. We have found no quick fix for muscle-based pelvic pain. A slow, deliberate rehabilitation is what we have observed in successful treatment.

TRIGGER POINT RELEASE AND THE RELEASE OF EMOTIONS

Sometimes during the course of internal trigger point release, deep emotions related to the tightness in the pelvis come to the surface. These emotions are often related to feelings that have been suppressed in relation to some kind of trauma or significant emotional event. Grief, fear, and anger sometimes arise, and these can occur.

It is important to understand that the release of these emotions (they don't always occur) is part of the resolution of the condition being treated. It should be looked upon positively. There is nothing to be alarmed about when these emotions arise. People usually feel a sense of relief after these experiences. Sometimes it is appropriate to explore these emotions in psychotherapy as a way of resolving them.

PREPARATION FOR *TRIGGER POINT RELEASE*

The self-treatment trigger point release sessions are best regarded as special times that need to be protected from the demands of the outside world. For this reason we suggest that, when possible, the patient do self-treatment physical therapy sessions in a relaxed way at a time when the patient has no responsibilities afterward. When possible, we suggest bathing and doing a relaxation session focusing on feeling and accepting the sensations that are present after the trigger point release session.

THE IMPORTANCE OF REGULAR
SELF-TREATMENT

The experience, understanding, and intuitive talent of a physical therapist guiding and supervising trigger point release can make the difference between success and failure of our protocol and the reduction or resolution of one's symptoms or not. But the most exhaustive physical therapy done brilliantly, while essential in our protocol, cannot guarantee that the offending trigger points will behave.

Consider that there are 168 hours in a week. Let us say that a person goes to see the physical therapist two times a week. That is quite a bit of physical therapy. In the physical therapy session, after you take off your clothes, give the physical therapist a report on your week, and begin the physical therapy itself, at the most you get probably thirty to forty-five minutes of hands-on treatment. After the treatment, the tissue is stretched (although sometimes temporarily irritated in the process). At the level of two appointments per week that is, at the most, one and a half hours of therapeutic treatment per week. In a good pelvic floor physical therapy session, the pelvic floor tissue has been lengthened, trigger points have been deactivated, and life has been made more livable for it.

After such a session, however, patients often experience what could be called "the parking lot phenomenon." In the treatment of muscle-based pelvic pain, for instance, you go into the parking lot after a physical therapy session, get into your car, get on your cell phone, and get back into your life. Your partner is upset about something on the phone, your work calls with a problem, traffic is bad, and your body's same protective guarding and tension, part of your default mode of tension, easily reasserts itself. A good physical therapy session can be reversed in an hour of bad traffic.

The resolution of pelvic pain is an inside job of cooperating with the healing requirements of the pelvis.

After physical therapy twice a week, there are approximately 166 hours remaining in the week to live. The old habit of going one hundred miles an hour in one's life and tightening up the pelvis regularly and squeezing and shortening the irritated tissue and interfering with its healing, as we have discussed, can easily and quickly undo the therapeutic impact of the physical therapy session. This is why it is necessary to engage in a program of ongoing regular relaxation of the pelvic floor and quieting of the nervous system with a relaxation protocol like the one we use, in close connection with regular daily physical therapy self-treatment that repetitively loosens the tissue. Trigger point release is an essential component of treatment but, in our experience, for most people is not sufficient by itself. Furthermore, pelvic pain syndromes, even when they do go away, can come back during periods of stress. Knowing how to treat yourself and not having to run to a professional, in our view, makes the flare-up far easier to face and deal with.

THE TRIGGER POINTS AND
THEIR REFERRAL SITES

Let us move on to a more detailed discussion of trigger point release. Drs. Janet Travell and David Simons introduced trigger points to modern medicine. Their first edition of *Myofascial Pain and Dysfunction: The Trigger Point Manual* in 1983 was the culmination of research that went back to 1942 when Dr. Travell published her first article on myofascial pain. Travell is well known for having been appointed the White House physician during the Kennedy and Johnson administrations. She was given this position as an expression of Kennedy's gratitude for her successful treatment of his myofascial pain that so affected his life and political career. We are fortunate that our senior physical therapist, Tim Sawyer, who has been the architect of the physical therapy aspect of our protocol, studied closely with Travell and Simons and then treated patients with them for years.

The concept of trigger points is relatively new to medicine. It is very new to urology. Trigger points are defined as taut bands within a muscle, either at the surface of the muscle or inside the muscle, in the belly or the attachment of the muscle. The trigger point characteristically elicits a twitch response, detectable on ultrasound or via electromyograph (a machine that measures the electrical activity in a muscle in millionths of a volt). The trigger point response can be felt by a trained and sensitive practitioner while palpating the trigger point. When the trigger point is pressed there is often a "jump" response in the patient, due to the reflexive reaction of the patient to the often exquisite tenderness of the trigger point upon palpation. Furthermore, the trigger point characteristically refers pain/sensation to the site being pressed or to a site remote from it.

A trigger point can be active or latent. An active trigger point is considered able to refer pain and re-create that pain upon palpation when the patient comes in with a complaint of pain. A latent trigger point has the capacity to be the source of pain and under certain circumstances to become an active one, but generally the patient does not complain of symptoms from latent trigger points. Trigger points are latent in many people.

Where one feels the pain is often not the source of the pain. For this reason the diagnoses of pelvic pain by doctors unfamiliar with the workings of trigger points are often mistaken because they are unclear that the source of much pelvic pain is not where it seems to be. While the concept of referred pain is well understood in medicine, the idea that pelvic pain felt in the groin, penis, testicles, vagina, or perineum may originate in a trigger point inside or outside the pelvic floor is far less readily understood. The difficulty that doctors have with trigger points is that they have usually received no training in the subject. Furthermore, because there is no objective, litmus paper, gold standard test for evaluating them, the only way clinically to find and treat them is through skillful palpation. This requires training and a sensitive touch.

A woman called us who had very severe rectal pain. She reported that during one of her doctor's pelvic exams he hit a spot that, the woman said, "sent me through the roof." After the exam, the doctor told her that he really did not know what was going on with her, that he couldn't help her and she might simply have to live with the pain. The woman went home despondent, her pelvic floor very irritated and flared up. The next day she woke up and her pain was almost gone. It remained so for several days. She called up the doctor's office happily bewildered to share with the doctor what happened. She told the nurse that she thought it was related to the painful spot the doctor pressed. The nurse relayed the news about the woman to the doctor. The doctor then told the nurse to tell the patient she could massage that point herself if it helped her. The patient felt more bewildered.

What probably happened is that the doctor inadvertently pressed and temporarily released a major trigger point for the woman and the woman responded much as any of our patients typically respond—with some flare-up and then a reduction of symptoms. The doctor, in not understanding trigger point pain and treatment, essentially dismissed this event and the possibility of helping this woman. His ignorance may have had a profound effect on his patient, as the experience left her confused.

Trigger points can refer pain that is directly on the trigger point site to a remote site, which means that where you feel the pain is often not where it actually is coming from. For instance, we find that tip-of-the-penis pain is often referred from trigger points in the anterior portion of the levator ani muscle as it attaches to the prostate. This is not obvious and is counterintuitive. This trigger point is a good five inches from the tip of the penis. Who would think that the source of tip-of-the-penis pain would be a site so relatively far away? To complicate matters further, if you do not have long enough fingers or if you do not understand how the trigger points work in the body, you miss this connection entirely. And if you don't keep pressure on an internal trigger point for the length of time we know is necessary, the trigger point remains active.

The internal muscles that contain trigger points are close to each other, and it takes someone who understands the internal pelvic anatomy and is experienced in feeling the muscles inside the pelvic floor to tell them apart.

All of the muscles, both internal and external, must be evaluated and treated. When muscles are known to contain trigger points referring pain to an area that the patient is complaining about, they should be examined carefully. The therapist must be trained in identifying trigger points and must be able to feel for superficial and deep trigger points located in the belly and the attachments of the muscles. Most importantly, when trigger points are located, they must be held with pressure release and other release techniques according to the "pressure principle" we formulated. When appropriate, the following techniques are used:

- Voluntary contraction and release/hold-relax/contract-relax reciprocal inhibition
- Spray and stretch occasionally with stubborn external trigger points
- Deep tissue mobilization, including striping, strumming, effleurage
- Myofascial release/skin rolling
- Strain-counterstrain/muscle energy release

Anyone who has pelvic pain of the kind we treat should know that specific trigger points in specific pelvic muscles tend to refer specific kinds of symptoms. This knowledge is critical for the physical therapist who is treating pelvic pain and training patients in self-treatment. As we have mentioned, pain in the tip of the penis or the sense of urgency and frequency is typically created by active trigger points in the anterior (front) portion of the levator ani muscle as it attaches to the prostate. When the physician or physical therapist does an examination, knowledge of the relationship between symptoms and pelvic trigger points is essential to making the diagnosis of muscle-based pelvic pain and dysfunction. We are much more confident in our diagnosis and ability to help the patient when we find relationships between the trigger points and the kinds of symptoms they typically refer.

*Trigger points can release after the beginning
sessions of treatment. What often remains is sore,
contracted tissue that can take many months
or longer to restore to soft, pain-free tissue.*

Trigger points are sometimes idiosyncratic, and not all patients fit all the patterns we describe here, so they must be located manually. Sometimes only one or two trigger points fit the referral pattern we describe below. Importantly, we sometimes can help people with tight and tender pelvic muscles where we find no discernible trigger points.

INTERNAL PELVIC FLOOR TRIGGER POINTS IN MEN AND WHERE THEY TYPICALLY REFER PAIN AND SENSATION

In working internally, we generally place patients in the prone position with a cushion under their stomach. The right hand is used to examine and work the left side of the pelvic floor and the left hand to work the right side of the pelvic floor. Patients tend to feel less vulnerable and more comfortable in this position, and it affords the practitioner good access inside and outside the pelvic floor.

The illustrations on pages 76–81 show trigger points in the internal pelvic muscles.

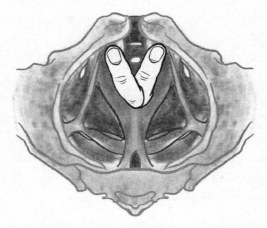

Anterior Levator Ani, Superior Portion (or Puborectalis)

This is one of the most important trigger point sites in male pelvic pain, and palpating high enough up and firmly enough is critical in proper treatment. Frequently this area is the site of trigger points that are responsible for the tip-of-the-penis and shaft-of-the-penis pain. Furthermore, trigger points in this area can refer to the bladder, urethra, pressure, and fullness in the prostate.

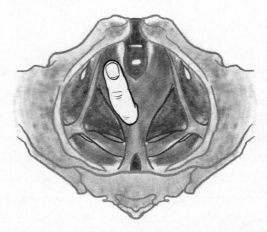

Anterior Levator Ani, Middle Portion (or Levator Prostate)

Trigger points in this area can refer pain and pressure to the base of the penis, prostate, bladder, and pelvis and re-create frequency and urgency.

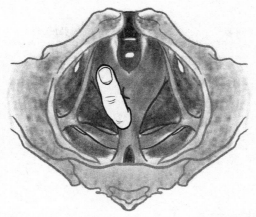

Anterior Levator Ani, Inferior Portion (or Puborectalis)

Can refer pain and pressure to the perineum, the base of the penis, and the prostate.

This is one of the most common and important trigger points in male pelvic pain.

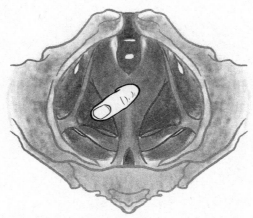

Middle Levator Ani (or Iliococcygeus)

Trigger points in the middle levator ani (iliococcygeus) typically refer lateral wall pain, perineal pain, and anal sphincter pain. Trigger points can refer forward toward the anterior levators and the prostate. Trigger points here can refer discomfort associated with a sense of prostate fullness.

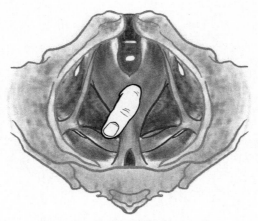

Coccygeus/Ischiococcygeus

Trigger points in this muscle typically refer pain and pressure associated with the sense of having-a-golf-ball-in-the-rectum, pain to the coccyx, and gluteus maximus. Pre– or post–bowel movement pain is often associated with the sense of having a full bowel.

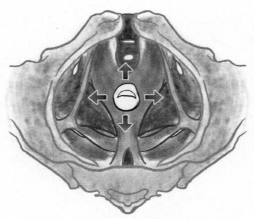

Sphincter Ani

Trigger points in this area may cause anal pain in the anal sphincter itself as well as pain going toward the front and back part of the anal sphincter. Treatment is done by gently stretching the sphincter upward in the 12 o'clock position, sideways in the 3 o'clock position, downward to the 6 o'clock position, and sideways toward the 9 o'clock position.

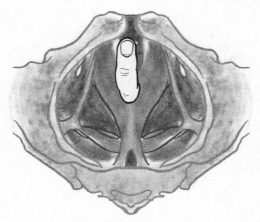

Prostate Massage Area

Traditionally urologists massage the prostate to extract prostatic fluid in order to examine it under the microscope or to drain the prostate of inflammation or infection. The massage of the prostate in the *Wise-Anderson Protocol* is not done for this purpose. We massage the prostate when the physician specifically prescribes this massage, or we do it to stretch the associated connective tissue. While some physicians do prostate massage vigorously or roughly, we do not. Especially if the prostate is tender, we are very gentle at first and our purpose is to desensitize the sensitivity of the prostate so that with repeated ongoing massage over a period of a number of massages, the prostate becomes less painful. Our method of prostate massage is as follows: We locate the prostate and do lateral sweeps from outside to inside when the finger is on one side (lateral to the medial) of the prostate. And then from the other side with either hand, we do lateral to medial (outside to inside) sweeps . . . always going from the outside to the center of the prostate. We then go from the top to the bottom (superior to inferior). If the prostate is excruciatingly painful, we are particularly gentle. The duration of the entire massage is approximately one minute.

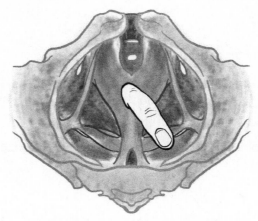

Piriformis (internally accessed)

Trigger points here can refer to the sacroiliac joint, the hip girdle, and hamstrings. Patients can feel increased pain at the palpation site.

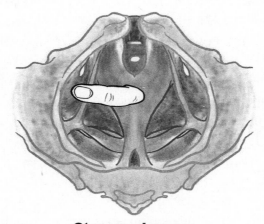

Obturator Internus

Trigger points in the obturator can refer pain to the perineum, outward toward the hip, or to the whole pelvic floor, both anteriorly and posteriorly. The obturator is intimate with the pudendal nerve and can refer a dull ache and burning in the pelvic floor on the side on which it is being palpated. Trigger points in the obturator can refer the golf-ball-in-the-rectum feeling, symptoms to the coccyx, hamstrings, and posterior thigh. In women, trigger points in the obturator can refer to the urethra, the vagina, and specifically the vulva and is a very important point in the treatment of vulvar pain.

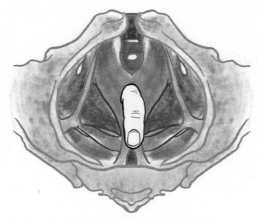

Palpating the coccyx

This is a bony palpation. In treating pelvic pain, if the coccyx is immobile, it can be a factor that perpetuates trigger points that cause pelvic pain.

External Pelvic Floor Trigger Points and Their Referral Sites in Men

External trigger points can be as important in perpetuating a pain cycle as internal trigger points. For example, we treated a man for whom significant groin pain came from his quadratus lumborum muscle, located on the side of the body. Again, this trigger point was relatively far away from where the pain was felt. When this trigger point was treated, the man experienced tremendous relief. Every doctor that this man saw in the years he suffered with this trigger point missed this. We have treated people who have had abdominal trigger points that refer excruciating pain into the pelvis.

To the therapist experienced in myofascial/trigger point release, the patient's symptoms and the physical examination give the essential clues as to the location of the trigger points.

The following illustrations show trigger points in the external muscles that can contribute to pelvic pain.

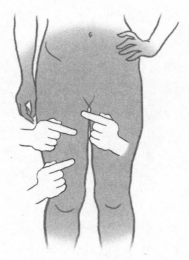

Adductor Magnus

This muscle is missed by many clinicians.

The adductor magnus is a critical muscle to check for trigger points that can refer pain throughout the pelvic floor, including the perineum, bladder, and prostate.

When trigger points continue to be active internally, the culprit may be unresolved trigger points in the adductor magnus.

Trigger points in the adductor magnus can refer the sensation of having a golf ball in the rectum.

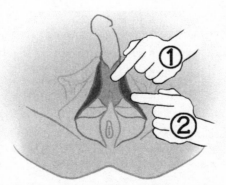

1. Bulbospongiosis and 2. Ischiocavernosis

Trigger points in the bulbospongiosis and ischiocavernosis can refer pain and sensation to the base of the penis and perineum.

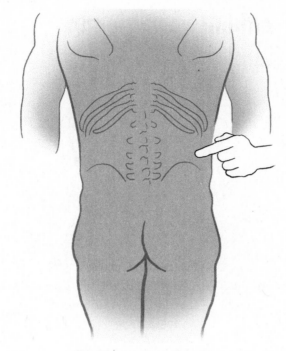

Quadratus Lumborum

Crest of the ilium and the lower quadrant of the abdomen.

Outer aspect of the groin (can refer to labia in women, testicle or lateral penis in men)

Greater trochanter (hip) and to lateral upper thigh

The sacroiliac joint

The lower buttock

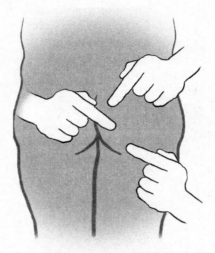

Gluteus (Maximus)

Trigger points in the gluteus maximus can refer pain and sensation into the hip buttocks, tailbone, sacrum, and hamstrings.

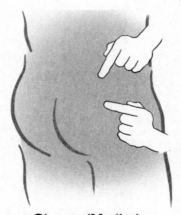

Gluteus (Medius)

Trigger points in the gluteus medius can refer pain and sensation around the buttocks, hip girdle, and down the leg as well as into the testicles.

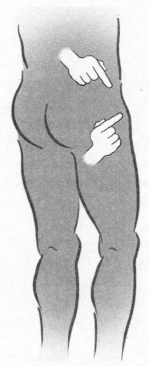

Gluteus (Minimus)

Trigger points in the gluteus minimus can refer pain and sensation down the leg and sometimes into the testicles.

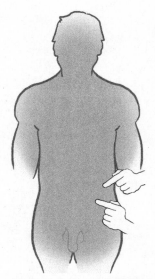

Lateral Abdominals Oblique

Trigger points in the lateral abdominals can refer pain to the whole stomach, up into the ribs, down the groin, and into the testicles. This is an important source of testicular pain.

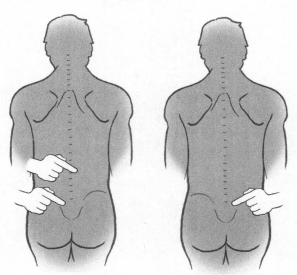

Paraspinals and Multifidi

Trigger points in the paraspinals tend to refer pain and sensation into the low back; however, this is pain that doesn't tend to fan out but is tightly contained in a specific area.

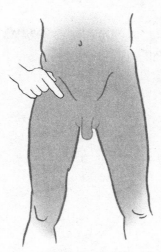

Pectineus

Trigger points in the pectineus can refer pain and sensation to the groin. This is a major trigger point for groin pain.

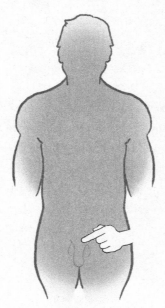

Iliopsoas

Trigger points refer to anterior thigh and groin.

INTERNAL AND EXTERNAL PELVIC FLOOR TRIGGER POINTS AND THEIR REFERRAL SITES IN WOMEN

On the following pages we have compiled the internal and external trigger points most frequently implicated in pelvic pain in women.

   The illustrations on this and the following pages show trigger points in the internal and external pelvic muscles.

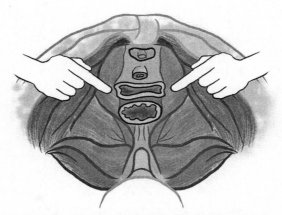

Anterior Levator Ani (Inferior Portion)

This is the part of the muscle closest to the back of the pubic bone. Trigger points can refer to the bladder, urethra, clitoris, mons pubis, vaginal lips (labium majus and minus), or vestibule (entrance) of the vagina. Trigger points referring discomfort to the bladder can be associated with a sense of urinary urgency.

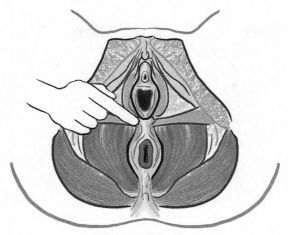

Perineal Body

Trigger points in the perineum can refer pain and sensation to the rectum, vagina, and site of palpation.

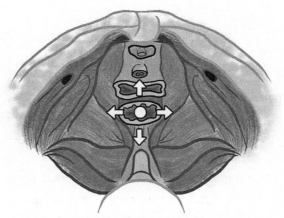

Sphincter Ani (Stretch)

Trigger points in this area may cause pain in the anal sphincter as well as pain going toward the front and back part of the anal sphincter. Treatment is done by gently stretching the sphincter upward in the 12 o'clock position, sideways in the 3 o'clock position, downward to the 6 o'clock position, and sideways toward the 9 o'clock position.

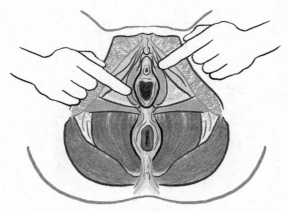

Bulbospongiosis and Ischiocavernosis

Trigger points in the bulbospongiosis and ischiocavernosis can refer pain and sensation to the perineum and vagina.

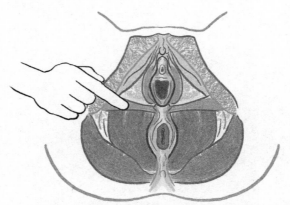

Superficial Transverse Perineal Muscles

Trigger points in the superficial transverse perineal muscles can refer pain and sensation to the vagina and on the site of palpation.

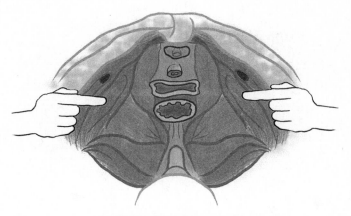

Obturator Internus

Trigger points in the obturator can refer pain to the perineum, outward toward the hip, to the whole pelvic floor, both anteriorly and posteriorly. The obturator is intimate with the pudendal nerve and can refer a dull ache and burning in the pelvic floor on the side that it is being palpated. Trigger points in the obturator can refer the golf-ball-in-the-rectum feeling symptoms to the coccyx, hamstrings, and posterior thigh. In women, trigger points in the obturator can refer to the urethra, the vagina, and specifically the vulva and is a very important point in the treatment of vulvar pain.

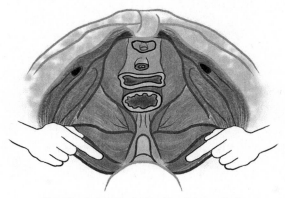

Piriformis (Internally Accessed)

Trigger points here can refer to the sacroiliac joint, the hip girdle, and hamstrings. Patients can feel increased pain at the palpation site.

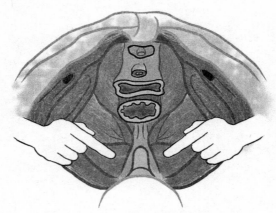

Coccygeus—Ischiococcygeus

Trigger points in this muscle typically refer pain and pressure associated with the sense of having a golf ball or stick in the rectum, or pain to the coccyx, anus, and gluteus maximus. Pre– or post–bowel movement pain is often associated with the sense of having a full bowel.

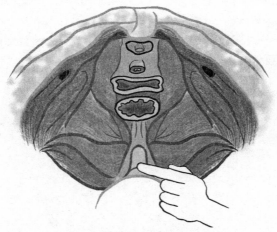

Palpating the Coccyx

This is a bony palpation. In treating pelvic pain, if the coccyx is immobile it can be a factor that perpetuates trigger points that cause pelvic pain.

WISE-ANDERSON PRESSURE PRINCIPLE

One of the most important things we teach at our immersion clinic is a technique for doing internal pelvic floor trigger point therapy. This technique has come from our years of experience in working with the internal tissue and it is called the *Wise-Anderson Pressure Principle*. We have taught the tenets of the *Wise-Anderson Pressure Principle* to our patients since the beginning of our work, referring to it with different conceptual language at different times, such as "greeting the pain." We now give it a more formal name emphasizing its importance.

The *Wise-Anderson Pressure Principle* is one of the most important things we teach to our patients related to internal trigger point release. We take this opportunity to discuss the details of the *Wise-Anderson Pressure Principle,* especially in relation to the tendency in some patients to become overly aggressive in conducting their own self-treatment. Importantly, this issue is highly relevant to patients just beginning our protocol because the internal tissue tends to be the most sensitive when one first starts the internal self-treatment. However, the *Wise-Anderson Pressure Principle* remains of critical importance throughout the entire arc of the self-treatment program.

It is our view that myofascial restriction and the presence of trigger pointed muscles have existed for years in most pelvic pain patients we see, and bring perspective in understanding the *Wise-Anderson Pressure Principle* to tread very lightly in internal trigger point release

From the beginning of our work, we have based our treatment on the understanding that pelvic pain is closely associated with the muscles of the pelvic floor being in a state of what variously can be described as protective guarding, chronic contraction or hypertonus, typically in response to anxiety and importantly in response to uncomfortable or painful tissue irritation pursuant to chronic pelvic guarding. In most patients, we believe that this state has typically occurred for a very long time, often years or even decades in some patients. Restoring the pelvic muscles to a normal, noncontracted state can be uncomfortable at first.

Imagine how sensitive your gums would be if you were brushing your teeth now for the first time.

The purpose of this internal self-treatment is to permit the healing of the chronically irritated and guarded pelvic tissue into relaxed and supple and pain-free tissue, like the pelvic tissue of someone without pelvic pain.

Sometimes the pelvic floor muscles may feel bewildered that you are asking them to change their level of tension and their guarded behavior. Some pelvic tissue triggers dysfunctional protective guarding. Indeed, especially in the first months of doing the protocol, the internal tissue tends to continue to be very sore and tender, and sometimes *any* contact with the tissue may temporarily increase discomfort. Thus, in the *Wise-Anderson Pressure Principle* technique we describe below, the goal is to find a "sweet spot" pressure level in each patient that allows for a gentle, competent palpation of the restricted tissue while avoiding being overly aggressive in a way that could be irritating to the tissue. This is a balancing act that requires close attention and intention on the part of the patient. By paying careful attention to finding the Pressure Principle "sweet spot," we have observed in many cases that the patient can maximize the effectiveness of their self-treatment and at the same time reduce the possible flare-up of symptoms.

The *Wise-Anderson Pressure Principle* technique is as follows: once the patient has gently inserted a generously lubricated gloved Internal Trigger Point Wand or finger, the finger or Wand simply rests inside without pressing on any tissue. The patient just feels the presence of the finger or Wand inside the anal sphincter or vaginal opening while applying no pressure. This gentle, stress-free time is to help the pelvic floor and internal anal sphincter or vaginal opening adapt to having the finger or Wand inside; it is what we call the "neutral position." Indeed, there are pelvic pain patients who suffer from such a tender or sore pelvic opening that just resting with the finger or Wand inserted, and not pressing in any particular direction, can be a sufficiently therapeutic stretch of the tissue for the first few months or so of self-treatment.

With the Wand or finger in the neutral position, the tip of the Wand or tip of the finger is then pressed against a specific restricted area of tissue. Pressure with the finger or Wand stops at the moment that one begins to experience an intimation of pain or discomfort. In other words, pressure remains at this level without eliciting any increased discomfort. This minimal static pressure that elicited the beginning awareness of pain or discomfort from the tissue is considered the "sweet spot" that we referred to above. This is the *Wise-Anderson Pressure Principle*. With our patients at our immersion clinics, we usually recommend maintaining this minimal static pressure against the tissue for 30 to 90 seconds, depending upon the circumstances of each patient.

The "sweet spot" level of pain or discomfort may or may not dissipate quickly during the internal self-treatment, but pressure is not increased if it occurs.

Sometimes, the pain or discomfort response elicited following this principle dissipates after the static pressure is applied (it usually takes at least fifteen seconds before this to begin when it does occur). If the tissue releases and no longer produces pain/discomfort, the pressure may cease to be exerted or it can be gently maintained for a little longer in order to encourage the lengthening that has occurred.

When the patient is ready to move on to another trigger point or area of tenderness, we first suggest that the Wand tip or finger rest inside for a moment in the neutral position, not pressing in any direction. Close attention needs to be maintained as self-treatment continues. If one is in pain or anxious, it can take a few seconds for any pressure to consciously register.

Over time, as the trigger point and restricted tissue resolves its irritability, more pressure is typically required to elicit the same pain or discomfort on tender, contracted internal tissue.

By using this *Wise-Anderson Pressure Principle* technique, we have observed that most patients are able to exert more pressure on the tissue to elicit the same level of discomfort as weeks and months go by. Following this method of gradual and non-traumatic progressive pressure, it is rare for the patient "to get out ahead of the tissue" or to try to force his/her own timeline of healing on the tissue. Using this technique, the internal tissue is the "guide" as to how hard to press. This is the practice of *listening* to your body.

Our research has shown that, in regard to internal self-treatment, pressing harder does not mean more symptom improvement. Awareness of the sweet spot of the initial threshold of pain or discomfort, from our experience, is the best way to help the tender, contracted pelvic tissue out of its contracted state. Patience with and sensitivity to the internal tissue is key. The principle to follow: kindness to the internal tissue, listening to it, being guided by it, working with it, not imposing anything on it that unduly irritates it. The *Wise-Anderson Pressure Principle* helps the internal tissue not dread internal treatment.

We always suggest incorporating therapeutic assistance around internal treatment, like hot baths for those whom heat helps in order to help keep the area calm and soothed. This principle allows the internal tissue to be the guide and tell the patient how hard to press. These are the themes of the *Wise-Anderson Pressure Principle*.

EXTERNAL TRIGGER POINTS RELATED TO FEMALE PELVIC PAIN

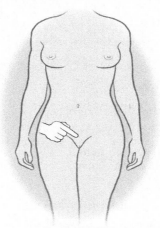

Pyramidalis

The pyramidalis is not present in some individuals, but when it is present and has trigger points, they can refer pain and sensation to the bladder, pubic bone, and urethra.

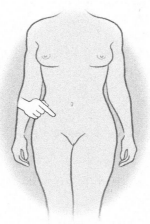

Iliopsoas

Trigger points in the iliopsoas can refer pain to the groin, labia, anterior (front part) thigh, and low back.

When constipated, passage of stool can trigger pain.

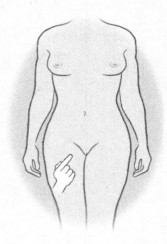

Pectineus

Trigger points in the pectineus can refer pain and sensation to the groin. This is a major trigger point for groin pain.

Sexual activity that involves vigorous squeezing of the thighs can activate these trigger points (especially in women).

Adductor Magnus

This muscle is missed by many clinicians.

The adductor magnus is a critical muscle to check for trigger points, which can refer pain throughout the pelvic floor, including perineum, rectal, or vaginal pain (and less often bladder pain).

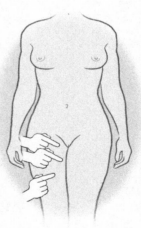

Deep groin pain, which is sometimes described as generalized internal pelvic pain.

Patient has difficulty identifying pain in any specific pelvis structure.

Pain over the pubic bone.

Pain sometimes described as shooting up inside the pelvis.

Sometimes symptoms occur during sexual intercourse.

When trigger points continue to be active internally, the culprit may be unresolved trigger points in the adductor magnus.

Trigger points in the adductor magnus can refer the sensation of having a golf ball in the rectum.

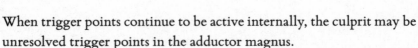

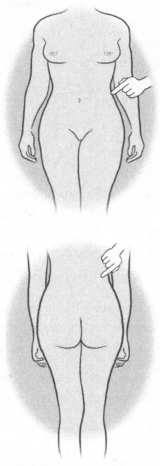

Quadratus Lumborum

Trigger points in this muscle are one of the most commonly overlooked muscular sources of pelvic pain. It is a complex muscle made up of both deep and superficial fibers, which refer pain to the sacroiliac region, hip, buttock, abdomen, and groin.

In the female patient, pain can also be referred to the anterior thigh, labia, and vagina.

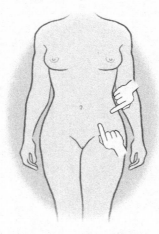

Lateral Abdominals Oblique

Trigger points in the lateral abdominals can refer pain to the whole stomach, up into the ribs, down the groin, and into the vagina and labia. This is an important source of vaginal and labial pain.

Gluteus (Maximus)

Trigger points in the gluteus maximus can refer pain and sensation into the hip, buttocks, tailbone, sacrum, and hamstrings.

Can refer pain to the entire buttock and tenderness deep within the buttock.

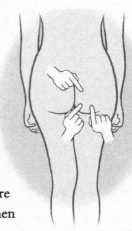

Can refer pain that covers the entire lower sacrum.

Sitting on a hard seat can feel like a nail is pressing into the sitz (or sitting) bone.

Pain in the coccyx (coccygodynia).

Restlessness or pain on prolonged sitting (more than 15–20 minutes) and increased pain when walking uphill or swimming crawl stroke.

Needs to sleep with pillow placed between knees; sit upright on soft surface (not donut or in slouching position).

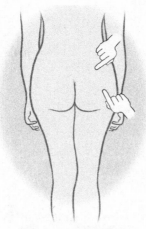

Gluteus (Medius)

Trigger points in the gluteus medius can refer pain and sensation around the buttocks, hip girdle, and down the leg as well as into the vagina.

Sometimes is the cause of hip pain in later stages of pregnancy.

Needs to sleep with a pillow placed between knees and in side—lying on unaffected side (rather than on back); sit upright on soft surface (not donut or in slouching position).

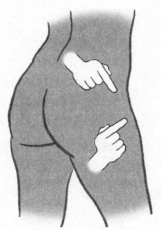

Gluteus (Minimus)

Trigger points in the gluteus minimus can refer pain and sensation down the leg and sometimes into the vagina.

Some of these trigger points are found through deep palpation.

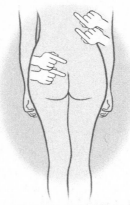

Paraspinals and Multifidi

Trigger points in the paraspinals tend to refer pain and sensation into the low back; however, this is pain that doesn't tend to fan out but is tightly contained in a specific area.

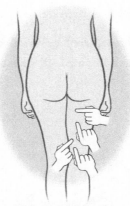

Hamstring Muscles

Trigger points in the hamstring can refer pain to the back of the leg down to the back of the knee.

The gluteal crease and the ischial tuberosity (may cause difficulty sitting).

Can be associated with trigger points in the obturator internus, piriformis, and gluteals.

Can also be confused with sciatica.

DIFFERENT METHODS OF
TRIGGER POINT RELEASE

Many who wish to follow our protocol are confused about how to tell what is or is not useful physical therapy and training in self-treatment. Our perspective comes from working with many patients who have seen us at Stanford with whom we have used the *Wise-Anderson Protocol* over the years.

We have interviewed many patients who have seen a variety of physical therapists. We have listened carefully to the comparison of their experiences with physical therapists we know are competent in our protocol and their previous experiences. To sum up, *not all physical therapy for pelvic pain is the same or is effective.*

Modern medicine can be likened to Christianity and schools of thought in medicine to the different denominations like the Baptists, Unitarians, and Episcopalians. In the world of physical therapy, there are different churches or schools of thought about how, for instance, you do trigger point release. Our protocol closely follows the methods of Travell and Simons. Many patients that we have seen have been treated previously by physical therapists using different methods. They have shared their experiences and compared them to our protocol and the others they have used.

> *We are convinced that the methodology*
> *we use is by far the most effective in the*
> *treatment of patients with trigger points.*

Here are some important points about the *Wise-Anderson Protocol* for physical therapy of the pelvic floor. Perhaps the most important point is that the skillfully trained patient, with the right equipment, is their best myofascial trigger point therapist. If trigger points are not palpated vigorously and specifically enough, the trigger points can simply resist deactivation. Yet there is danger of injuring the tissue if the pressure is inappropriately vigorous. We discuss this in the *Wise-Anderson Pressure Principle*. Experience and talent in feeling the tissue and sensing how much to palpate are imperative. Physical therapists who are not experienced in dealing specifically with pelvic pain and training patients in self-treatment may err in several ways—most importantly, they do not find the trigger point, they are not vigorous enough in palpating when the trigger point is found, or they do not use pressure release on the trigger points for thirty to ninety seconds.

Flare-up of symptoms is common especially after the first trigger point release sessions. These flare-ups usually abate as treatment continues, although they can recur. Without this knowledge, we have seen some inexperienced therapists back off from treatment after a patient's flare-up out of fear that they did something wrong. Their concern immediately gets across to the patient, who becomes concerned about going down the wrong road. Doubt about physical therapy and the whole course of treatment arises, and it is not uncommon for patients to stop treatment.

When people do trigger point release, it is best, when possible, to not immediately go back into a situation of demand and tension. Think about the physical therapy that we do as a stretching and lengthening of contracted tissue that can allow it to rest and heal; taking time after a therapy session to remain quiet and rest the pelvic floor is important. A tightened pelvic floor is usually the physical expression of a psychologically defended state, and releasing the pelvic tissues can trigger emotional release and psychological insight during or after the physical therapy session.

The management of expectations in trigger point release self-treatment is essential: both that flare-ups are common and to be expected and that progress often occurs over a span of many months. Often treatment can feel like three steps ahead and two steps back for quite a while. The idea that there should be a quick fix represents a misunderstanding about the healing of sore pelvic tissue. It is important to understand that the healing of pelvic floor irritated tissue, in the midst of a busy life, requires self-treatment that encourages and coaxes the tissue to relax and lengthen. The pelvic floor doesn't respond to force or a hurry-up-and-get-better attitude.

We have defined what we include in our protocol and what we do not. A summary is provided.

- The emphasis of our physical therapy work with pelvic pain is on trigger point release. We consider a thorough examination of possible interior and exterior trigger points to be essential in our protocol. Our protocol is most promising when we can find internal or external trigger points that tend to re-create a patient's symptoms. It should be said that while we have the most consistent success with people in whom we can find trigger points that re-create their symptoms, sometimes we have helped people with no clear trigger points but with a much-contracted pelvic floor.

- Pelvic floor biofeedback is a process in which an anal probe is inserted and the patient is asked to do EMG-monitored Kegel exercises. At this point, as a rule we do not use pelvic floor biofeedback therapeutically. Also, we consider unremarkable pelvic floor biofeedback readings a poor measure of what is going on in the pelvic floor or whether our protocol is indicated.

- Generally, we do not use electrical stimulation either at the office or for home treatment and have not found it useful.

- In our view, myofascial release alone is not an adequate treatment for pelvic floor pain. If postural and/or mechanical factors appear related to the pelvic pain, we treat the most important perpetuating factors found, including postural obliquities. We treat posture and pelvic obliquities often and instruct patients in relevant home stretches and/or stabilization exercises. If the postural perpetuating factor is large, we refer the patient to a physical therapist closer to his or her home.

- *Skin rolling or connective tissue massage* can be an important self-help tool that many of our patients are encouraged to use. This method is explained on the next page.

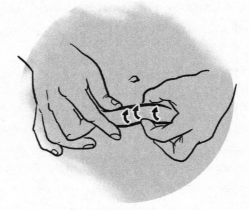

Skin Rolling

It is difficult to explain how to do skin rolling. It is not simply a pinching of the skin and rolling it in place, but rolling the skin while moving the roll of skin downward just as a wave moves from off shore to the shore. Skin rolling is rolling the skin down or up in a moving wave. The point is that in skin rolling, you roll the skin downward, sideways, or vertically but the skin roll isn't stationary—it moves. In other words, you alternatively walk the fingers along the skin by continuously pushing down with the thumb and up with the index and third fingers and thereby move downward, rolling the skin as the skin rolls move downward.

- We train our patients to do home *Trigger Point Release* using our Internal Trigger Point Wand, our new Trigger Point Genie, and some other tools.

- We generally do not do prostate massage. From our perspective, the purpose of prostate massage is to stretch the associated connective tissue especially where it attaches to the prostate, and not to drain prostatic fluid.

- While we appreciate the efficacy of Feldenkrais, craniosacral manipulation, the Alexander method, internal Thiele massage, and other modalities for many kinds of problems, we generally do not use or recommend these methods for the pelvic pain we treat.

- Before and after treatment, we use gentle, moderate, or deep effleurage or Swedish-type massage on the external areas (gluteals, back, legs, and stomach).
- Our physical therapy protocol is based on the knowledge that multiple trigger points can refer to one place and that each trigger point must be evaluated and treated.
- We use pressure release of trigger points, applying pressure for up to ninety seconds.
- We encourage patients to self-treat both internally and externally after proper supervision.

HOME STRETCHING PROGRAM

The muscles of the pelvic floor are easily contracted, but stretching them in the way that you can stretch your shoulders or arms is not so easily accomplished. However, they can be stretched to some degree. We consider it essential to train patients in relevant stretches and ask patients to perform these several times a day throughout the week. They include stretches of the adductor and pectineus muscles, the lateral rotators and piriformis, the iliopsoas muscle, the quadratus lumborum, the hip abductors, and the abdomen.

We educate our patients in doing diaphragmatic breathing while doing these stretches. When possible, we encourage patients to take a hot bath and then do external trigger point release before stretching.

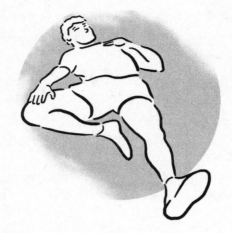

1) Pectineus Stretch

Do this stretch while lying down on your back on a firm surface and first bending one knee while resting the other unbent leg on the floor. A hand is placed on the same side as the bent knee on the inside of the knee and then the knee is slowly pushed outward toward the floor and held for fifteen to thirty seconds.

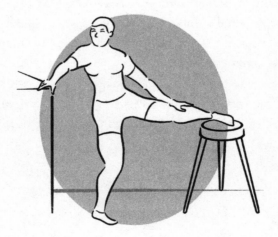

2) Adductor Stretch

In this stretch, bend slightly the knee that is supporting you in order to increase or decrease the stretch on the inner thigh. The leg is stretched out on a stool and held for thirty seconds or longer. The leg changed after one adductor is stretched to stretch the other adductor. We do not do this stretch if any pain in the knee is experienced.

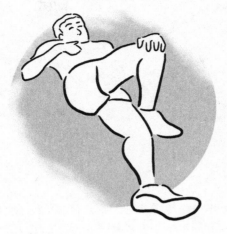

3) Lateral Rotators/Piriformis Stretch

This stretch is done lying down on the back on a firm surface. As in stretch #1, the knee is bent while resting the other leg unbent on the floor. This stretch is held for fifteen to thirty seconds and can be done daily.

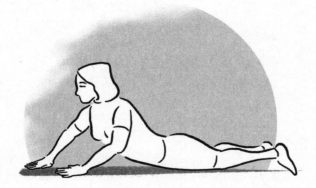

4) Cobra

This is a well-known yoga stretch done on the stomach while slowly pushing the upper body upward by straightening the arms and bending back the lower back.

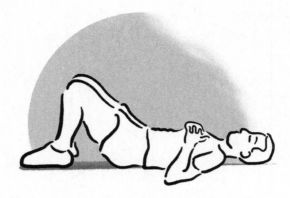

5) Pelvic Tilt

This stretch is done on a firm surface, face up with both knees bent. The abdomen is tightened with the buttocks, with the result of rocking the pelvis and putting the lower back flat against the floor.

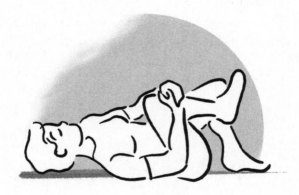

6) Knee Pull

This exercise is done on the back on a firm surface. Both knees are bent with the feet resting comfortably on the floor.

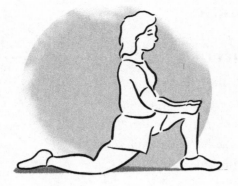

7) Kneeling Stretch of the Iliopsoas

This exercise is done kneeling on one leg with the other leg pulled back. With the upper body vertical and erect, without bending the head forward, the body is shifted forward, stretching the thigh and groin for five to twenty seconds.

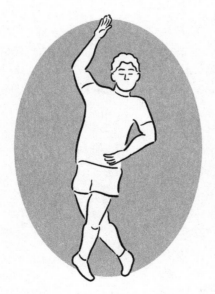

8) Stretching the Quadratus Lumborum and Hip Abductors

This exercise is done standing with the hands on the hips. One leg is crossed in front of the other.

9) Squat Stretch

This stretch opens up the pelvic floor. The squat is done on both feet with the back supported against the wall without your "sit bones" touching the floor. When there is no discomfort, this position can be held for one minute or longer, depending on the advice of a physical therapist or physician.

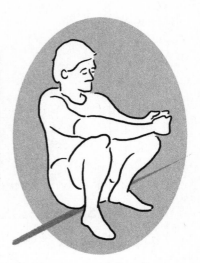

SELF-ADMINISTERED TRIGGER POINT RELEASE

In the *Wise-Anderson Protocol* we teach people how to do both internal and external trigger point release on themselves, whether manually, with a tennis ball, with a Trigger Point Genie (described below), or, for internal points, with our FDA-approved Internal Trigger Point Wand.

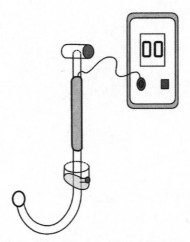

Internal Trigger Point Wand

THE *WISE-ANDERSON* INTERNAL TRIGGER POINT WAND WINS FDA APPROVAL

Since we began the development of the *Wise-Anderson Protocol* at Stanford University Medical Center in the department of urology in the mid-1990s, we recognized the need for a special device to do internal trigger point release self-treatment for those with muscle-based pelvic pain. After a multi-year, large clinical trial and a rigorous approval process, the Internal Trigger Point Wand, designed by David Wise, won FDA approval in 2012.

Our Internal Trigger Point Wand is the first FDA-approved scientifically designed device for patient use in doing internal myofascial/ trigger point release related to pelvic pain that has been scientifically tested in a clinical trial, and whose results have been published by a peer-reviewed journal and presented in scientific meetings. In our study published in 2011 in the *Clinical Journal of Pain*, the median reduction in sensitivity/pain of trigger points after 6 months of self-treatment reported by patients with pelvic pain moved from 7.5 to 4 on a 1-to-10 scale. This is a remarkable result. In our experience, we have observed that trigger point sensitivity and symptoms associated with them continue to drop in many of our patients as they continue to use our protocol after six months.

We have presented the Wand at the International Continence Society in San Francisco in 2009 and at the American Physical Therapy Association Meetings in New Orleans in 2011; the results of our Wand study were presented at the American Urological Association meetings in Washington in May 2011. The abstract on our Internal Trigger Point Wand won an award at the American Urological Association meetings, was presented to the public in a press conference sponsored by the AUA, and was nominated for presentation at the AUA meetings in Tokyo.

WAND HISTORY

When we began seeing patients from out of town at Stanford University Medical Center, like other practitioners, we thought conventionally about treatment of pelvic pain. Patients came to us for treatment and the participation of the patient in the essential internal trigger point release part of our program, aside from the relaxation protocol, in large part was passive: internal trigger point release was done on them by physical therapists. We referred our local patients to physiotherapists for weekly or biweekly internal trigger point treatment and the physiotherapists would do physical therapy on them. We found some therapists seemed to be of little help and a few seemed to have excellent results. At that time, we consistently received reports of outstanding results from patients seeing Tim Sawyer, who is our senior physical therapist. When we consulted with Dr. David Simons, the coauthor of the original trigger point release book with Janet Travell, he told us that Tim was the best trigger point therapist in the country. Tim brought his extensive expertise and talent to our program and over the years designed what we consider the best training in self-treatment for patients that exists.

Before the Wand, we attempted to help patients who lived far away to find physiotherapists and coach the physiotherapist in internal trigger point release. When it was possible, we attempted to teach the partners/spouses of our patients how to do internal physical therapy. This sometimes seemed a better option than referring them to physiotherapy, because there was no cost in partner-administered internal trigger point release, and because treatment could be done more frequently and more conveniently.

Partner-administered internal trigger point release, however, was not perfect. It tended to be hit or miss as to whether a patient had a partner, and whether the patient was willing for a partner to do pelvic floor physical therapy on him/her. As important, it was not uncommon for a patient to be reluctant to have an intimate person do something so bold as internal trigger point release. Finally, we could only teach a partner rudimentary skills and the patient and partner were limited by the narrow competence of the partner.

The Internal Trigger Point Wand has been a major advance in our treatment of pelvic floor dysfunction and allows patients to do their own internal trigger point release easily, comfortably, and without cost.

Over the years we have developed a training protocol that is part of our six-day immersion clinic, which centrally includes careful training and supervision in the use of the Internal Trigger Point Wand. When we teach our patients to use the Wand, we consider it critical for them to understand the practice of internal trigger point release and internal myofascial release. If one does not understand what the point of trigger point release is, both internally and externally, and if one is not instructed in the proper method of identifying trigger points and areas of restriction, the frequency of use, and the proper pressure to use on them, self- treatment typically founders.

The area inside the pelvis is foreign territory to most people. Quite understandably, most people have never put their own finger up inside their anus or vagina as you must to do internal trigger point release. It is not surprising that there can be shame, fear, and bewilderment about doing what would appear to most people as a very strange thing. When our patients begin to feel the pain reduction and relief of symptoms that accompanies this activity when done for the purpose of releasing trigger points and painfully constricted tissue, any feelings of aversion to this activity quickly disappear. Our patients soon realize that the inside of the pelvis is just another part of the body that can hurt, and whatever relieves the pain in the pelvis is welcomed as a gift and a blessing.

The Internal Trigger Point Wand frees trained patients from having to consult with a physician, physical therapist, or other practitioner to do competent and effective internal trigger point release self-treatment. It allows patients to comfortably and at no cost do regular internal trigger point release, including internal trigger point release where a therapist is not able to reach. Anterior trigger point release is easily and comfortably done on the back. There is a pressure gauge that displays relative pressure remotely so no pressure-reading device needs to to be inserted inside the pelvic floor. A movable stop limits the insertion of the Wand and assists with navigation inside the pelvis.

Most important, we have had years of experience in training patients to use the the Internal Trigger Point Wand. Simply inserting an object in the pelvic floor without any instruction often results in a flare-up of symptoms and the patient who has no idea what they are doing inside, or where they are with an object inserted inside, ceasing to do internal trigger point release out of an anxiety about what they are doing. Doing internal trigger point release with our Internal Trigger Point Wand is done by a patient only after careful training and supervision.

THE TRIGGER POINT GENIE AND EXTERNAL TRIGGER POINT RELEASE

External trigger point release is typically done on the abdominals or muscles above the pubic bone, the adductors or the muscles of the inner thigh and around the perineum, the gluteal muscles (minimus, medius, and maximus), the quadratus lumborum, and other external trigger points associated with pelvic pain. The program of self-administered external treatment for pelvic pain was developed by Tim Sawyer, our senior physical therapist. One should rely, not on the instructions for the kind of trigger point release described here, but on the instruction and supervision of a physical therapist knowledgeable in this technique.

Using the Trigger Point Genie

On the following pages we illustrate the use of the Trigger Point Genie in working with some external trigger points related to pelvic pain. The Trigger Point Genie is a device that makes it possible to do trigger point release in a way that has not been possible before. Most trigger point tools focus pressure on a trigger point using a hard plastic, wood, or metal tip that is often uncomfortable and does not allow relaxation while applying the pressure against the trigger point. The Trigger Point

Genie uses comfortable rubber balls to enable relaxation while pressure is exerted by the ball tip.

Components of the Trigger Point Genie

The purpose of the Trigger Point Genie is to use the weight of the body on the rubber ball and with a chosen length of threaded rod to apply specific pressure on a particular trigger point while resting on a comfortable surface.

Pressure can be applied with more or less force to a sore muscle or trigger point in the body. Resting the part of your body that is going to be placed on the ball of the Trigger Point Genie allows gravity to exert pressure. The ball of the Trigger Point Genie is gradually rested on to increase the amount of pressure being exerted on the trigger point.

The purpose of the different-sized rods is to do trigger point release comfortably in different places in the body illustrated below, with specific comfortable pressure.

The purpose of the different-sized ball/tips is to be able to specifically target tight muscles in the body of various sizes that require different focal pressure.

USING THE TRIGGER POINT GENIE FOR EXTERNAL TRGGER POINT RELEASE

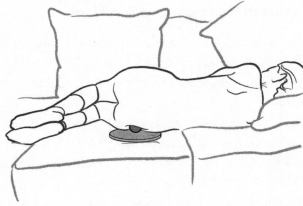

FIG. 1

Releasing trigger points in the *gluteus minimus*, *medius*, and *maximus* by resting on a tennis ball against a wall.

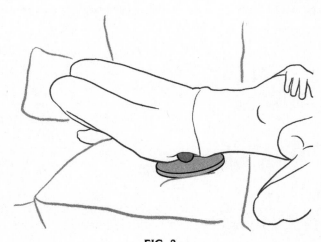

FIG. 2

Identifying the *gluteus minimus*.

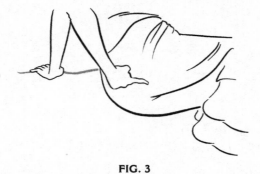

FIG. 3

Identifying and doing trigger point release on *gluteus maximus*.

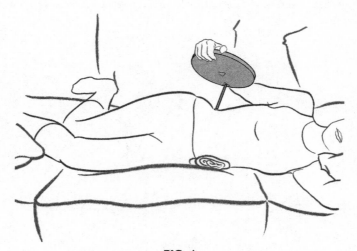

FIG. 4

Using the Trigger Point Genie to release
***quadratus lumborem* trigger points.**

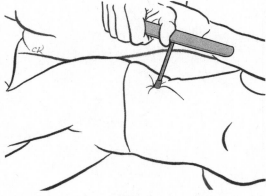

FIG. 5

Using the Trigger Point Genie to release quadratus trigger points. Care must be taken to not press on the twelth rib.

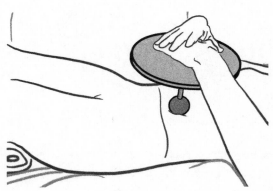

FIG. 6

Using the Trigger Point Genie to release
rectus abdominus **trigger points.**

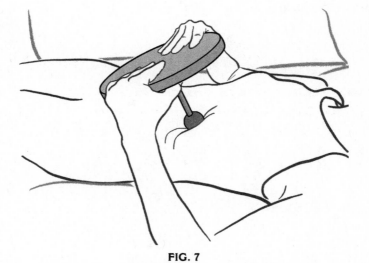

FIG. 7
Releasing trigger points in the abdominals.

USING THE TRIGGER POINT GENIE FOR ABDOMINAL TRIGGER POINT RELEASE

The best leverage we have found in using the Trigger Point Genie, our latest device for doing external trigger point release when doing abdominal trigger point release with the Genie, it is very important not to put undue pressure against the aorta in the middle of the abdomen; the instructing and supervising physical therapist should show the patient where this is in the midsection, a little to the left in the abdomen, and how to avoid putting pressure on it.

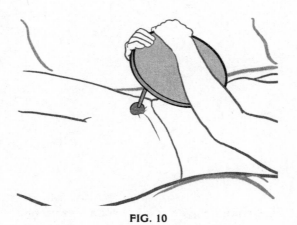

FIG. 10

Releasing trigger points in the *iliacus* using a Trigger Point Genie.

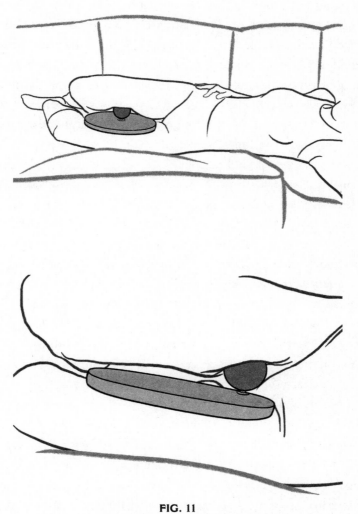

FIG. 11
Releasing trigger points in the *adductors*
using the Trigger Point Genie.

Many pelvic pain patients have increased muscle tension and trigger points in the large muscles of the hip girdle. They can treat these areas by stretching, leaning on a tennis ball against the wall, or later using the Trigger Point Genie. Tim Sawyer has noticed, however, that many therapists and patients overlook important potential trigger points in the middle and lower areas of the buttocks around the greater trochanter and the "sit bones" (or ischial tuberosity). These muscles include the lower part of the gluteus maximus, the piriformis, and other short lateral rotator muscles of the hip (gemelli, quadratus femoris, and the obturators and the proximal insertion of the adductors and hamstrings).

Patients who continue to struggle with different aspects of sitting pain, tailbone, rectal, and perineal pain, visceral pain that some men describe as deep prostate pain, back of leg pain, and hip pain may be overlooking the role that trigger points can play in these muscles. We encourage our patients to develop the confidence to use their fingers or Genie to explore these small, important muscles for painful trigger points and areas of tenderness and restriction, and then to treat these areas repetitively with either gentle massage using olive oil or massage lotion, a ten- to fifteen-second milking/strumming technique, or a fifteen- to ninety-second pressure-release technique. Often trigger points and areas of restriction and tenderness in these lower-buttocks muscles can feel "nervy" or "tingly" or very sensitive to the patient and this can prevent or scare the patient from treating these areas. If any of these sensations are experienced during our clinic or after, we ask our patients to check in with our physical therapist before proceeding.

Trigger points in these lower hip girdle and upper leg areas, however, have been known to cause troubling types of pain and uncomfortable sensations. Having the confidence to return to them again and again with appropriate pressure and proper treatment often enables the release of the trigger points and restriction in these muscles. When these muscles are untreated they can play a perpetuating role in both external and internal pelvic pain and dysfunction.

In doing trigger point release self-treatment,
it is best to start gently and slowly increase
in terms of vigor used on the tissue.

APPLYING THE *WISE-ANDERSON*
PRESSURE PRINCIPLE EXTERNALLY

Generally we have found in our work that the externally accessed muscles are less sensitive and/or less inclined to irritations or flare-ups than the internally accessed pelvic floor muscles. Of course, if there are significant flare-ups or irritation after doing external release, then the patient is probably pressing too hard (see the "Hyperirritability" section below). For this reason it is best for patients to listen to their tissue and allow it to be their guide.

If patients find they flare up their external tissue, we suggest they be guided by that first elicitation of pain/discomfort, as described above with regard to using the *Wise-Anderson Pressure Principle* for internal self-treatment.

Trigger points should be pressed only to
the beginning of discomfort and not so
hard that one is in agonizing pain.

In our experience, the trigger point, to be deactivated, has to be pressed to the point of the beginning of discomfort but not overwhelming pain. If we were to quantify pressure on a scale of 0 to 10, where 0 is none and 10 is the most extreme, in general the internal trigger point should be pressed at the level of approximately 1, the very first sense of discomfort. We ask patients to simply "greet the pain" at a level of 1.

Trigger points should not be pressed so
lightly that there is a complete absence
of discomfort upon palpation.

If the trigger point is pressed with great force, causing an amount of pain that one cannot relax with triggering protective guarding, the trigger point will tend not to release. This kind of forced trigger point release is sometimes done by men and women who think that they have to power through their pain and bear the consequences. But such overly aggressive self-treatment, in our experience, is counterproductive and usually fails.

> *Trigger point release should not be done*
> *so hard that the patient cannot relax*
> *while the trigger point is palpated.*

For best results, the patient must feel sufficiently safe and trusting to at least begin to relax during the pressure. Pressing on a trigger point when the patient is resisting the pressure instead of relaxing with it isn't a good idea.

Some patients have reported that if they can't relax with the pressure, then their trigger point usually doesn't let go. This is telling and intuitive. We want to be firm but gentle and sensitive with ourselves in all ways. Trigger point release has to be a cooperative and relaxed dance between the recipient of the trigger point pressure and the pressure on the trigger point.

When the patient is beginning to use the protocol to self-treat external trigger points, we encourage him or her to not go beyond a 3 subjective pressure level. Like internal therapy, external trigger point release is a process of "coaxing" the tissue out of a tightened state and into a relaxed, supple, pain-free state; the goal is not to try to get rid of the symptoms in any one trigger point session. Trying to do this usually results in the patient being too aggressive and unnecessarily irritating or flaring the muscles up. Daily, repetitive coaxing is the rhythm and concept we are going for—not imposing a time line of healing on the tissue but listening to the tissue and allowing it to be the guide.

HYPERIRRITABILITY

In this vein, we want to discuss the phenomenon of pelvic floor hyper-irritability. Some patients are so sensitive and have such a high level of pelvic tissue irritability that one cannot touch their anal sphincter or vagina or even lightly press on any related trigger points without causing excruciating pain. This hyperirritability is crucial to understand and work with.

> *Hyperirritable trigger points can calm down
> and release over time with patience, work,
> and a kind and accepting attitude.*

When hyperirritable patients work with themselves, they have to proceed carefully. We instruct patients to do gentle skin rolling on their abdomen, inner thighs, and perineum preceded and followed by long soothing strokes, massaging these muscles. We encourage them to do this before they do any work close to the genitals or anus. Putting warmth on these areas or taking a warm bath is useful in conjunction with the skin rolling and the long-stroke massage of the abdomen and the inner and outer thighs and buttocks.

Hyperirritability will usually accommodate to increasingly greater pressure on the trigger point if the level of pressure is very gradually increased over a period of a number of weeks or months. This has to be done with an attitude of kindness toward the body and trust that the body wants to get better and be free of the pain.

> *The reality of treating the condition of muscle-
> based pelvic pain is that it took a long time for the
> tissue to get the way it has gotten and it has its own
> timetable for healing. Patients who do well tune in to
> their own bodies and cooperate with this timetable.*

Trigger point release should not be done with the idea that you can "hit a home run" and knock out the pain quickly. There is no race here. There must be no urgency to get rid of the pain. One must be patient and bring the body along with graduated levels of stretching and discomfort in pressing on trigger points. We are quite happy if patients trained in self-treatment have to take three to twelve months or longer of regular skin rolling, self–trigger point release, and stretching to calm down their hyperirritability. Any other attitude that contains urgency and insensitivity in doing the physical therapy component of our protocol is counterproductive and tends to stall treatment. Hyperirritability may also be caused by an underlying perpetuating factor that only a skilled therapist or MD who understands and treats myofascial pain can evaluate.

ADDRESSING PELVIC PAIN REQUIRES *BOTH* EXTERNAL AND INTERNAL SELF-TREATMENT

Patients inexperienced in our protocol often think that if they are in pain inside the pelvis, the only place to treat the internal pain is inside the pelvic floor. As a result, they exclusively focus on the internal treatment. This is a common mistake among patients and physical therapists, so let us be absolutely clear: the external muscles are usually intimately involved in internal pain and must be treated along with the internal tissue. The adductors, abdominals, psoas, iliopsoas, quadratus lumborum, and gluteal muscles, with variations in each patient, are typically all part of the complex regional myofascial restriction creating internal pelvic pain.

Patients trained in our protocol are taught to comprehensively treat these external areas in addition to performing internal treatment. In fact, in certain cases, we have seen some patients significantly reduce or even resolve what felt like solely internal pain by treating trigger points and restriction in the external muscles listed above. Simply focusing on the internal trigger points and areas of restriction to treat internal pain to the exclusion of the related external trigger points represents a misunderstanding of the problem and often leads to a stasis in treatment.

The *Wise-Anderson Pressure Principle* represents an understanding of what contracted and trigger-pointed tissue inside (and outside) the pelvic floor needs in order to loosen, relax, become supple, and heal. Incorporating this principle in a self-treatment program is slow going and requires the development of patience, perseverance, commitment, and an understanding of the tenets of our protocol. It is a practice of listening to the body and being guided by the tissue, and not overriding the tissue's natural time line of healing with one's own aggressive, incorrect concept about how long healing should take.

CHAPTER 4

THE *WISE-ANDERSON PROTOCOL*, PART 2: EXTENDED PARADOXICAL RELAXATION (EPR)

(This chapter was written in the first person by David Wise.)

From all of my teachers, I have grown wise
Psalm 119

In developing *Extended Paradoxical Relaxation,* I stand on the shoulders of those with whom I have studied: Edmund Jacobson, Jean Klein, Jim Simkin, Hakuun Yasutani, Erik Peper, Larry Bloomberg, Alexander Lowen, and Alan Leveton, and those whose work I have studied: Roberto Assagioli, Fritz Perls, Byron Katie, Nisargadatta, Ramana Maharshi, Philip Kapleau, and others.

One of the most important influences in learning relaxation came from my study with Edmund Jacobson, considered the father of relaxation therapy in the United States. His method, *Progressive Relaxation,* has been used in one form or another throughout much of the twentieth century. Many research studies have been done on the effectiveness of *Progressive Relaxation* in treating conditions ranging from constipation to ringing in the ears. Despite much misunderstanding about Jacobson's method, even among professionals who use it, *Progressive Relaxation,* as Jacobson practiced it, has stood the test of time.

I was fortunate to have met Dr. Jacobson in 1977 at a conference in Chicago of researchers using his method. It proved to be a turning point in my life, as *Progressive Relaxation* became the starting point for me to develop what I have called *Extended Paradoxical Relaxation,* which I used in my own recovery from pelvic pain and in my development of the method to help my patients who found themselves in pain and anxious and otherwise unable to quiet down.

Jacobson was born in 1888 to a middle-class family in Chicago. A brilliant student, he graduated from Northwestern University in two years. At age eighteen he attended Harvard University. He taught physiology at the University of Chicago and later went to Rush Medical College, where he received his M.D.

It is known that when he was eight years old, a fire broke out at an apartment house owned by his parents. Tragically, a close friend of theirs was killed in the blaze, and Jacobson's parents became distraught over this shocking loss. The level of their distress deeply disturbed young Jacobson. He reported later in life that at the time of the fire he'd vowed never to get upset the way his parents had. This desire to remain calm and relaxed stayed with him through adolescence.

Later, when dealing with his insomnia as a Harvard undergraduate, he began to experiment with his own methods of relaxation. As he developed a technique that allowed him to sleep, he chose to write his doctoral dissertation on an experiment showing that tense subjects responded acutely to a stressor (two metal bars clanging), while subjects trained in relaxation hardly reacted at all.

Jacobson devoted his life to applying the principles he developed in *Progressive Relaxation* to the treatment of many psychosomatic disorders. In 1924, he treated women with globus pharyngis (archaically known as globus hystericus), a condition in which the patient feels that there is something stuck in the throat. Jacobson documented the narrowing of the esophagus in this condition by capturing images of the esophagus with a fluoroscope. He then trained these patients in *Progressive Relaxation* and 'scoped the esophagus again afterward. Not only were the subjective symptoms resolved, but the fluoroscopic images of barium, ingested in order to visualize the contours of the esophagus, also verified a widening of the constricted portions of the esophagus.

For decades, Jacobson treated a variety of conditions with *Progressive Relaxation*—a treatment few of his time could understand. He successfully treated hypertension; spastic esophagus; spastic colon; headache; functional cardiac disorders such as esophageal spasm, heart palpitation, and arrhythmia; as well as the gamut of psychological problems, including anxiety disorders, depression, and mania. He documented the effectiveness of relaxation treatment in the many studies he published. Perhaps more remarkable is that Jacobson proposed the link between stress and illness decades before it became fashionable. It is also noteworthy that while he helped his patients when no other treatment did, he conducted scientific research into the subject of the relationship between body and mind in the conventional medical remedies of the time. He wrote his classic book *Progressive Relaxation* in 1929 and then republished a revised version in 1939.

In the mid-1940s, Jacobson looked for a way to independently verify the efficacy of his method, that *Progressive Relaxation* actually lowered autonomic arousal and allowed patients to experience profound relaxation. At the time there were no reliable independent findings that could indicate whether someone was relaxed or whether there was any discernible change in nervous arousal as the result of Jacobson's intervention. In conjunction with Bell Telephone Laboratories, he developed the first electromyograph, an instrument able to detect electrical activity in muscles with a sensitivity of up to one millionth of a volt. With this tool, formerly undetectable physiologic effects could be easily and scientifically demonstrated. The electromyograph could objectively verify changes in muscle electrical activity whether someone was tense or relaxed, and the extent to which *Progressive Relaxation* impacted their psychoneuromuscular state.

Although the electromyograph formed the basis of the first of a number of different kinds of biofeedback machines, Jacobson did not incorporate the technological wonder he created as a tool in the clinical setting. He took the position that one could not learn to relax while looking at a meter or listening to a tone. He felt that the very act of looking or listening was tension producing and interfered with entering the profound states of relaxation he was aiming for.

As with anyone who teaches relaxation, Jacobson's method was one of attempting to teach the indescribable. He was clear that *relaxation required one to release effort*; that one learns to be consciously effortless in order for the nervous system to calm down. Jacobson's *Progressive Relaxation* is the practice of conscious effortlessness. His method was home-cooked and his language peculiar. He told his patients to "discontinue effort."

When I worked with Jacobson to learn to relax myself, he did not offer abundant detail to guide me through the inner terrain in search of stillness. The inner world we must spend our time in when we do relaxation is very subtle. Harivansh Lal Poonja, a meditation teacher, once told me that the most skillful of words can only point to, but cannot precisely capture, the subtlest aspects of what is the experience of inner peace. He said, "What it isn't can be described eloquently . . . what it is, is a kind of metaphorical room into which no words can enter." The same is true for relaxation training. The words can only point to what is not easily communicated in words.

THE EFFORT ERROR

One of Jacobson's important, and yet unheralded, contributions was his recognition that *effort cannot cease effort*. He emphasized this insight in his discussion of the *effort error*. He was a keen observer of minute tensions in the body that, when unrecognized, kept the nervous system aroused. He would observe patients doing relaxation and observe the subtle efforts, called muscle tension, that were invisible to anyone else.

His instructions and methods were didactic, authoritarian, and typical of the early twentieth century, reflecting the concepts of patient and doctor and student and teacher. Underlying his instruction was the unspoken edict that you scrupulously follow the teacher's instructions even though they tended to be terse and often obtuse. Jacobson's tendency to pay little attention to how his words might be received by patients and students, in my mind, is reflected in the only book of his that is currently in print, which he perplexingly called *You Must Relax*. If I did not know what kind of giant Jacobson was, a book with such a title, and its author, would have no credibility to me.

JACOBSON *WALKED THE TALK* OF HIS RELAXATION METHOD

Jacobson practiced relaxation daily for most of his adult life. Watching him do relaxation stunned me as I witnessed the effortlessness he displayed. In his writings, his public talks, and in my personal communications with him, he exuded a confidence in his understanding of nervous arousal, its role in a variety of stress-related disorders, that could only come from someone who lived and breathed and was the beneficiary of what he taught.

Edmund Jacobson practiced his own method. *Progressive Relaxation* was the first comprehensive relaxation system I know of whose developer actually walked his talk. One important limitation of his method, however, was his tendency to disregard the set of psychological experiences that students carry into the relaxation training session. Jacobson wanted to avoid having anyone confuse his method with reassurance or the transference of the patient toward the doctor that Freud focused on in psychoanalysis. Jacobson would tell his patients what to do without offering any reassurance or softness in style. I believe his terseness and lack of supportive language was an overreaction to his concern about the potential dismissal, invalidation, or trivialization of his method.

Finally, because Jacobson was very concerned that his method not be regarded as an offshoot of yoga, meditation, or spiritualism, his language in describing it and training someone in it tended to be mechanical and, for him, appropriate to the scientific and objective parlance of his peers. This language was sometimes not helpful, instructive, or accessible to those who read his work.

During Jacobson's time, medicine deliberately eschewed any religious or spiritual influence, and any hint that a method was spiritual or mystical made it suspect among the scientific illuminati of the time. Jacobson was careful to shun any hint that his method bore any relationship to so-called spiritual practices. In truth, the method of *Progressive Relaxation* is, in essence, in the finest tradition of the world's effective wisdom practices for bringing peace to body and mind.

PROGRESSIVE RELAXATION MISUNDERSTOOD

Ironically, Edmund Jacobson's method is best known for the least important instruction in his repertoire: to tense and then relax groups of muscles. Many who teach *Progressive Relaxation* misunderstand the method and think that tensing and relaxing muscles is its most important feature. This couldn't be further from Jacobson's intention. He told patients to contract and then relax the forearm, for instance, so they'd know how slight tension felt, and so they'd know what they were going to focus on and what they wanted to relax. The instruction to contract and relax muscle groups was most significant to those who were the least in touch with their bodies and could discern only very gross tension. The contract-relax instructions are aimed at the sensory reeducation of the least adept students of *Progressive Relaxation*.

Ultimately, what Jacobson called *residual tension* (the amount of tension that remains after one has *tried* to relax) was the key to relaxing nervous-system arousal. In teaching *Progressive Relaxation,* the teacher finds numerous students whose attention has been so routinely exteriorized that they have great difficulty even identifying the slight guarding, bracing, or tension that never relaxes.

Jacobson's method of focusing attention on one muscle group, using peculiar instructions like *discontinue effort, pull out the plug from the wall,* or *go negative,* was his best attempt to get his patients to practice consciously letting go of effort. Jacobson knew that focusing attention on certain parts of the body was more effective in achieving deep relaxation than focusing on other parts of the body. Relaxing the forehead, for instance, had a more calming effect on the nervous system than relaxing the arm.

The most profound part of Jacobson's method came from his discovery that the movement of the eyes is intimately involved in visual thinking (visualization), and the muscles of the speech apparatus, namely the lips, tongue, throat, jaw, and related muscles, are intimately connected to verbal thinking (subvocalization). He discovered that relaxing the eye and speech muscles permitted the practitioner to slow down or stop visualization and verbal thinking. In this slowing or cessation of thinking, in this "non-REM relaxation," which is a way I describe *Extended Paradoxical Relaxation,* the nervous system quieted profoundly and deep relaxation occurred. For some, relaxation of the eyes and speech muscles is key to their ability to quiet down.

THE ORGAN OF FEAR

Jacobson had a keen interest in the relationship between the reaction of the gastrointestinal tract, anxiety, and an aroused nervous system. He spent considerable time treating patients with what is currently called irritable bowel syndrome (IBS), but in his time was called spastic colon. He was also interested in the effects of relaxation and anxiety on the esophagus. When I first met him at a lecture he gave, I approached him afterward. In the course of our discussion, he told me that the esophagus was the "organ of fear." Jacobson felt that a relaxed esophagus and colon could not coexist with anxiety and an aroused nervous system.

Jacobson was the master of his method. A newspaper reporter who interviewed him toward the end of his life wrote that she acutely felt the level of her own nervousness through the mirror of being around such a profoundly calm man. The story goes that it was Jacobson's ability to relax deeply and reduce his metabolic requirement for oxygen that allowed him to comfortably stay underwater for several minutes.

WATCHING JACOBSON RELAX

I would never have learned relaxation had I not viewed it firsthand from Edmund Jacobson, the most ardent and passionate practitioner of his method. Forever etched in my mind is an evening meeting with Dr. Jacobson in the attic of his son's house in California. Jacobson looked at me and said, "I'm going to show you how I relax." Next, he said, "I'm relaxing my forehead and face now." Then he said, "Now, here go my neck, shoulders, arms, chest, back, stomach, pelvis, and legs." He did this in the course of a minute or two.

What stunned me as I looked at him in relaxation was that as he sat there, he looked like a corpse. Other than the muscles that held him sitting and the muscles of his heart and breathing, I saw no sign of muscle activity anywhere. His flesh just seemed to hang off his bones.

I found myself face-to-face with someone who was showing me what he was asking me to do.

The level of quiet I saw in him aroused the deepest feeling of wanting to be able to do what I saw him doing and have what I saw him having. To me, the miracle of it was that he was actually doing it—I'd found someone who was the real deal. In that moment, I saw that what Jacobson was teaching was possible. He demonstrated it effortlessly before my eyes. This personal experience was a rare gift in my life. It is so unusual in my experience to find the *real McCoy.*

As I recall Jacobson in that profound state of relaxation, it is clear to me that all the research he had done, the books he'd written, and his unflagging enthusiasm for his work were fueled by his daily experience of the energy and renewal that came from his regular relaxation practice. I understand this now because I see that the energy fueling my own work and writing fundamentally comes from my own experience of doing my own daily relaxation practice, during which I regularly experience profound relaxation and peace. Without the example of someone who really knew how to profoundly relax, I'd never have believed profound relaxation was really possible or committed myself to doing it as I have.

THE LIMITATIONS OF PROGRESSIVE RELAXATION LED TO *EXTENDED PARADOXICAL RELAXATION*

In my own struggle to learn to relax my own knotted-up pelvic muscles, I started in earnest with what I had learned from Dr. Jacobson. When I was with Dr. Jacobson, I often felt frustrated at knowing that he was the real thing and what he was able to do with Progression Relaxation was what I wanted to be able to do. But Jacobson's stinginess with words, and his reluctance to guide me verbally, were disheartening to me.

Over time, with the knowledge from observing him that convinced me that it really was possible to profoundly relax using a method, I discovered that one of the central keys to successful relaxation was to accept tension that did not relax. This struck me as a huge paradox: accepting what doesn't relax permitted me to relax. Accepting that I wasn't relaxed and not fighting it, disarmed the force inside me that kept me tense. In the presence of this paradox ultimately came the name *Extended Paradoxical Relaxation* for my revision of Jacobson's method.

In my many years struggling to find out how to relax, many insights came to me as I slowly gave up my preconceived ideas and instead remained open to my unfiltered experience. Here are some of my insights:

- I realized that being comfortable was hugely important for me in doing relaxation. This was at odds with the traditional meditation concept of sitting on an unsupported cushion, which I hated in the many years I practiced a variety of meditation methods. That I could fend off sleep in a comfortable position by periodically standing up and walking around when I felt drowsy was an important issue for me in choosing to be very comfortable doing relaxation instead of suffering with the discomfort of the traditional meditation posture.

- I realized that relaxation was easy. Babies were best at relaxation and they underwent no training. What became clear to me was not learning how to relax but instead how to manage the obstacles to being relaxed (i.e., my wandering mind, my pain, anxiety, negative thinking, my very need and sense of urgency to get somewhere and feel I was doing something) was what I had to figure out what to do with.

- I took Jacobson's seminal insight that the discontinuation of effort was the central task of relaxation (if you could call it a task), but only after years of work with this insight did I realize that there could be *no trying,* no attempt to change any sense of stasis in relaxation, *no trying* to discontinue effort if it didn't happen easily. Only those conditions offered an exit from the stasis and stuckness I would often feel.

- I realized that in accepting whatever was going on inside me allowed it to transform, and that acceptance had to include my resistance to this kind of acceptance.

- I realized that kindness to myself was the only thing that worked. When I became impatient, irritated, unhappy with myself, my progress and ability to relax regressed.

- I began to see clearly that what were called virtues in times past—virtues like patience, perseverance, kindness, surrendering impatience, and letting go of hankering after a quick fix to my suffering—were essential in my ability to calm down.

- What appeared startling to me was that my ability to focus my attention was the key to my ability to profoundly relax . . . something that actually seemed counterintuitive at one level to me.

- I realized that when I gave up trying to fix myself and get out of pain, and instead focused myself on accepting and resting with the condition I found myself in, that my condition improved and I was able to regularly reduce or stop my pelvic pain.

- In the state of inner calm, I noticed that my sore, irritated pelvis became less sore and eventually stopped being sore at all.

These and many other insights came to me as I became a sincere student of what helped my mind to focus and my nervous system to reset to states of peace and joy that I had only known as a child.

EXTENDED PARADOXICAL RELAXATION AND DISCOVERING THE DIFFERENCE BETWEEN A HALF-HOUR RELAXATION SESSION AND A TWO-TO-FOUR-HOUR SESSION

Years later, after a critical experiment, I observed that an extended period of time to do relaxation made a huge difference in the effects of reducing pelvic pain. After struggling with implementing this insight in my work with patients, I bit the bullet and began to ask patients to aspire to do two to four hours of relaxation at a time in a way I specified, until their symptoms were significantly better. While inconvenient and problematic in terms of many patients comfortably incorporating relaxation into their lifestyle, I have called this method of significantly extending the timeframe of doing Paradoxical Relaxation, *Extended Paradoxical Relaxation*. I consider *Extended Paradoxical Relaxation* a kind of healing chamber for the sore and chronically irritated pelvic tissue.

Historically, *Extended Paradoxical Relaxation* originated from our over twenty years of treating chronic pelvic pain patients using the *Wise-Anderson Protocol* for pelvic pain that we originally developed at Stanford University. Between 2005 and 2013, we published a number of scientific studies reporting our results in teaching our pelvic pain patients who have been refractory to any other treatment to use *Paradoxical Relaxation* and a specific myofascial/trigger point release method. With each year of our work over two decades we saw firsthand how essential *Extended Paradoxical Relaxation* was to calming down the autonomic nervous system and thereby their symptoms.

Extended Paradoxical Relaxation proved to be a breakthrough for us in which we've found that extending the length of time *Paradoxical Relaxation* qualitatively increased its effectiveness. In fact, it has been a watershed for many of our patients who have undertaken it. *Extended Paradoxical Relaxation* is done over an extended period of two to four hours at a time on a daily basis. And we are recommending that it be done for sixty days straight when the patient begins the practice. It can be modified and continued as needed after the first sixty days.

EXTENDED PARADOXICAL RELAXATION (EPR)

Extended Paradoxical Relaxation is the behavioral method that, in con-junction with a specific myofascial/trigger point release protocol, makes up the substance of the *Wise-Anderson Protocol* for the treatment of pelvic floor–related pain and dysfunction. The purpose of EPR is to provide a daily nervous system environment that will provide a regular heal-ing environment for the sore, trigger pointed and contracted tissue of and around the pelvic floor. Patients coming for training in the *Wise-Anderson Protocol* are trained in the practice of EPR and, after six days, are given a comprehensive recorded audio video program of *Extended Paradoxical Relaxation* lessons varying in length from two to four hours on a computer tablet that they take home and use on a daily basis in conjunction with pelvic floor physical therapy that they are trained in self-administering.

A way to describe relaxation at the deepest level is accepting what is-resting with what is. It includes acceptance of your aches and pains, your tension, your fidgetiness, and your resistance to letting go. The paradox is that when you give up trying to make something positive happen, that is when it is most likely to happen for you.

MORE ABOUT *EXTENDED PARADOXICAL RELAXATION*

- Relaxation needs to be done without distractions, but the most important thing is that one practices it regularly, even if the cir-cumstances aren't ideal.

- Relaxation is a time that is taken out for oneself where one need not respond to the various normal demands of life. It is a time in which you don't have to be "on." It's a time that is completely your time.

- A darkened room is easy to relax in. It is often helpful to use an eye pillow, which has the advantage of dimming the field of vision, even in a room with a lot of light. Phones are turned off, and the expectations are set with others in the household for the practitioner to not be disturbed during the relaxation time.

- We don't recommend listening to music or having the TV on. Nondistraction and physical comfort in *Extended Paradoxical Relaxataion* is essential.

- *Extended Paradoxical Relaxation* is the cultivation of effortlessness, not doing anything, including not exerting effort to breathe any particular way. It is resting in the present moment and just being at the most granular level.

- We sometimes suggest setting a timer at certain intervals during the extended relaxation sessions as a way of waking up and not staying asleep if one falls asleep.

- It is sometimes helpful to have a pen and a piece of paper nearby—a pressing thought can be written down so as to get on with the relaxation, undisturbed by trying to remember what the thought requires to be done.

- We encourage our patients to find the most comfortable body position—EPR can be done sitting or lying down. The tongue should be comfortable without any attempt to control it.

- Natural breathing—breathing should be easy and uncontrolled. Other than when our patients are practicing RSA (Respiratory Sinus Arrhythmia) Breathing, preparatory to an EPR session, we don't ask our patients to pay attention to the breath or control it. This is in distinction to other relaxation or meditation methods that focus on deep breathing or controlled breathing in order to relax.

- If one has an itch, we suggest you scratch it— if one feels like moving or fussing while doing relaxation, we suggest you simply move or fuss. Eventually the mind and body quiet down from such irritations.
- In *Extended Paradoxical Relaxation,* we focus on the slight, subtle sensation that occurs when one asks oneself to relax. Over and over.
- With great patience, perseverance, and earnestness we ask our patients to devote themselves to remaining focused. Controlled attention is the joystick of the nervous system, as we discuss.
- We ask our patients to not put themselves in "relaxation prison" with arbitrary, confining requirements to do this and not that. If our patients become fidgety and cannot relax, we suggest they stop and come back in five or ten minutes. If one can only relax comfortably for ten minutes, we encourage the patient to start with that.
- And, of course, we emphasize being safe. It is not advisable to practice this method of relaxation while driving, handling machinery, or doing anything that requires your full attention.

PRACTICAL TIPS AND UNIVERSAL STUMBLING BLOCKS EVERYONE FACES WHEN PRACTICING EPR

- Falling asleep during *Extended Paradoxical Relaxation* is more likely when one is tired, taking sedating medication, or doing the relaxation during a part of the day when one tends to become sleepy, such as in the afternoon or evening. EPR is not a nap. While it is not uncommon to fall asleep, especially if one is sleep deprived or taking a sedating medication, the issue of falling asleep can be successfully overcome.
- In my view, it is better to doze rather than to tense up for the purpose of staying awake. The experience of sleep during EPR tends

to be different from, and usually more beneficial than, simply falling asleep at night. As the relaxation proceeds into the second and third hour, alertness and focus tend to sharpen. The ten- to twenty-minute rule of fussing says that there tends to be period of fussing and distraction that usually occurs in the beginning of the relaxation session.

- It is often the case in doing EPR to go through a period of discomfort at the start of each session as you learn relaxation. Without persevering and getting past it, you can become discouraged and give up.

- How you deal with this period can determine how successful you become with EPR. It is helpful to be consciously aware of the fussing period that happens as you begin relaxation, and the often subtle discomfort and struggle to focus your attention during that time.

- I found that when I expected my relaxation to be immediate, not fussy, and uncomfortable, it took me longer to quiet down. That is why I think it is useful to accept this transition period in all its dimensions, to completely accept that it takes some time for attention to focus, for the body to settle, for your breathing to slow down, and generally to leave the state of activity for the state of being.

- Postponing caffeine until after an EPR session is generally advised.

Emotional Upset

- Sometimes we have a fight with a spouse or a friend or acquaintance, or receive an unwelcome notice from the IRS, or we lose our wallet, or find out that our job is in jeopardy. In cases like these, it is best, if possible, to process the upset before doing relaxation. It is usually best to talk to someone about it, make arrangements to solve the problem, or make a to-do list to at least organize your plan to deal with it. Once everything that can be done to remedy the situation is completed, then relaxation can start without the lingering distraction and anxiety.

When to Do Relaxation

- The best time to do *Extended Paradoxical Relaxation* is when you have the most energy. People usually find that they have this kind of energy in the morning. Some people have more energy and ability to pay attention in the afternoon. EPR requires energy because paying attention requires energy. Also, there are time constraints in many people's lives that dictate when relaxation can be done.

- It is best to regularly do EPR so the body gets used to a regular time of quiet. I advise people to do *Extended Paradoxical Relaxation* at least once a day for an extended period of time whenever possible.

- Many patients have hated doing relaxation in the beginning, because they hated the experience of being still and being present with what was going on inside them.

- After a while, however, most patients come to love relaxation and cannot wait to do it. Most realized that relaxation was essential to their recovery. This process of abandoning the relaxation regimen for a while and then coming back to it isn't abnormal.

- Many people succeed with EPR after they returned to daily practice. It is important to practice relaxation every day. If a session is missed, it can simply be made up. Hot baths, sauna, or other ways of warming the body are remarkable means of significantly reducing anxiety and nervous system arousal on a temporary basis.

- I can't be more enthusiastic about EPR. In my view, it is essential for the healing of a sore core of the body called pelvic floor pain. I love the experience of doing relaxation myself, and I do it not for pain but for the deepest enjoyment of my life. It revives me, calms me down, makes me able to be present with those I love and with the things I do every day. It is better than chocolate ice cream, and I love chocolatate ice cream.

Hot Baths

A hot bath is usually an effective if temporary means of lowering nervous-system arousal by itself. A hot bath, shower, or sauna can be particularly effective in preparing your body for *Paradoxical Relaxation*. Using heat has few side effects and is readily available and inexpensive. If heat helps lessen your anxiety, access to a hot tub—widely available at spas and health clubs—is a good idea. In the world of pelvic pain, a study demonstrated that a hot bath reduces the tension in the anal sphincter by one third. Even if the reduction of tension is short-lived, it is still pretty good.

DOING *EXTERNAL TRIGGER POINT RELEASE* USING THE TRIGGER POINT GENIE BEFORE EPR

For centuries, yoga practitioners have stretched the body with yoga postures (asanas) prior to doing shivasana, or a still pose in which meditation is practiced. Loosening the body can significantly help to jump-start relaxation and the ability to focus the mind. We give our patients an external trigger point release program of twenty minutes prior to doing EPR using the Trigger Point Genie.

*A thousand-mile journey begins with
a single step. Learning* Extended Paradoxical
Relaxation *begins with sitting or lying
down comfortably and focusing attention
on the slightest sensation of what relaxes inside.*

Taking the Long View and Managing Expectations

Though it might seem so in some cases, pelvic floor dysfunction doesn't come out of the blue. Someone can chronically tighten their pelvic muscles for years without symptoms, and then age or certain stresses trigger the symptoms. Just as those symptoms don't spontaneously appear, neither do they disappear overnight. Even with the most successful patients, it takes a significant amount of time for their symptoms to resolve. The body has often been in a state of chronic arousal for years. Finding a new way to exist in the world, without protective guarding ongoing states of fear, is not gained easily or quickly.

For those who are helped by this relaxation method, symptoms usually continue to improve (though flare-ups are common when stressful events occur) as people practice and gain mastery of this method over time. When this is done in conjunction with our physical therapy protocol, it can take considerable time for symptoms to reliably lessen.

Waiting three to six months to evaluate your progress doesn't mean that there won't be times when you feel better during or soon after you begin practice. Giving yourself this period reflects an understanding that most people's condition fluctuates, especially at the beginning of treatment.

Extended Paradoxical Relaxation Is a Practice—i.e., Something You Have to Practice to Get Good at It

To understand *Extended Paradoxical Relaxation,* you must understand that it is a "practice," something you practice. The word *practice* comes from the French *practiser* and from the Latin *practicare*. The term derives from the early fifteenth century, meaning "to perform repeatedly to acquire skill, to learn by repeated performance." When you practice something, you perform it repeatedly to acquire skill at what you are practicing. You learn by repeated performance of what you want to learn how to do.

It is easy to understand that you practice the piano for hours and hours to learn how to press on the piano keys in a certain way that produces a certain sound, and if you are reading music, you press on the keys in a certain way, timing your key pressing according to the instructions found in the music. You get good at pressing the keys in a certain way. When someone has practiced the piano for a long time, they play it well because they have played the piano over and over again. They get good at piano key pressing.

We know when someone has practiced the piano for a long time. We can hear it immediately. We can hear the lifetime of practice in a piano player like Artur Rubinstein. His skill is obvious. But what are you practicing getting good at when you practice *Extended Paradoxical Relaxation*?

EXTENDED PARADOXICAL RELAXATION IS THE SPECIFIC PRACTICE OF FOCUSING ATTENTION IN A CERTAIN WAY

We give our patients a comprehensive recorded relaxation course in *Extended Paradoxical Relaxation* to continue EPR practice on an ongoing basis after training in it at our clinic.

For someone who is interested in learning how to deeply relax and help heal a painful pelvis, understanding what I am saying here is really important. It is subtle. It requires a certain focus to understand the message I am communicating here.

If you want your body to deeply relax, you must find a way to control your attention so that your body is not continually stimulated by the stream of thoughts that typically go through your head. You must find a way to focus your attention on what does *not* arouse your nervous system. The most restful sleep, sometimes called stage IV sleep, occurs in dreamless sleep. If dreams are what we are thinking during sleep, the most restful sleep occurs when we are not dreaming (thinking) during sleep.

Now, the most quiet state for the body when not sleeping is simply to stop thinking. In practical terms, this doesn't mean to stop all thoughts from entering into our awareness. It means to focus attention away from thinking. When we are not focusing on thoughts that cause adrenaline to squirt into the bloodstream, the body quiets down. The environment that allows for healing comes about.

Extended Paradoxical Relaxation is a method that is best practiced between two to four hours per day in which you repeatedly shift your attention away from your thoughts and rest your attention in the subtle sensation of what is able to relax in you. The practice of focusing attention generally requires support from someone who is skilled in doing this. It is a subtle practice. In heroic sports movies when the baseball batter is shown in slow motion to be laser-focused on hitting the ball that sails into the home run stands, he has taken hold of his attention in that moment. In *Extended Paradoxical Relaxation,* we practice this laser focus in resting our attention in sensation. And when you can rest your attention in sensation, which is easier to do as you enter into the second, third, and fourth hour of EPR practice, the body quiets down and we enter into the healing chamber that occurs as the result of the control of our own attention.

> *Being good at controlling attention has huge*
> *consequences: beyond helping heal sore*
> *pelvic tissue, it can help you live longer.*

We all intuitively understand that prolonged stress can kill you or reduce your life expectancy. We all also intuitively sense that living peacefully probably helps your life expectancy. There are more than a few studies that show that people who meditate live longer and are healthier. Recent studies have shown that meditation affects the body on a cellular level by increasing an enzyme that is associated with longevity.

Extended Paradoxical Relaxation is a modern term for a certain kind of meditation for someone who is in pain and anxious. All meditation methods are methods of controlling attention in certain ways. The central practice of *Extended Paradoxical Relaxation* is controlling attention to rest in quiet sensation. In doing so, the nervous system can resume the default mode of a child: peaceful and happy, able to best heal what is sore and painful, having outsourced issues of survival to a loving parent.

The way in which you learn to control your attention in EPR opens the floodgates of insight and wisdom. Compassion toward yourself, the cultivation of patience, perseverance, acceptance, the existence of paradox in what is true, the experience that in letting go of what you want, it most likely comes to you, the experience that in doing what is best for yourself, you are most inclined to do what is best for others. . . . And on and on. The zone one can enter with the skillful practice of EPR is the zone one can enter with all real methods of meditation. And most important, learning to control attention so it is not hijacked by the unending stream of thoughts passing through awareness, can permit the experience of release of pelvic pain. And as a bonus it opens the doors to the experience of joy and peace that lies at the core of our being.

While returning your attention again and again to what relaxes inside when you ask yourself to relax, you practice accepting the intrusion of the smallest ache, the most ordinary feelings of unpleasantness, your inability to relax deeply, or your occasional or nonstop thinking, your losing your focus every other second. It is not that you dwell on any of the things you're accepting. Usually, you'll be aware of them briefly as they come into your awareness while you focus on the slight sense of *let go* in response to your instruction to yourself to relax. In EPR, you do your best to allow the intrusion of what is temporarily capturing your attention while returning your attention to the object of your focus without irritation or disappointment. You don't try to stop what is distracting you from occurring; you simply bring your attention right back to the sensation of your focus. *Extended Paradoxical Relaxation* is an inner experiment in staying focused on quiet sensation and un-reactively letting go of whatever intrudes on that focus.

Practicing EPR is like driving down a road where there are many sights and sounds. Your focus is on the road, but when something grabs your attention, whether pleasant or unpleasant, you bring your attention right back to the road without getting ruffled by what has momentarily intruded itself into your attention.

PROACTIVE ACCEPTANCE WITHOUT RESISTANCE TO ANYTHING

Doing *Extended Paradoxical Relaxation* is proactive, not passive. You're making a choice to focus while releasing your attention from everything on the periphery of your attention that comes into your awareness in the moment and tugs at your attention. You are asked to do this without any demand for gain, you just do it and then you observe what happens when you do.

> *If you feel like you're a mess inside, the*
> *best way out is to accept the feeling of the*
> *mess when it pulls at your attention.*

It is like falling into a mud hole and noticing that you don't want to get dirty. Then, finally understanding that getting dirty in such a situation is inevitable, you choose to surrender to being in a mud hole as you extricate yourself from it. You don't fight against the unpleasant feeling of the mud. In practicing EPR, you choose to focus moment to moment on what is most relaxed in your body while not resisting the messes of thought or other stimulii when they come into your awareness. You make a choice to un-reactively free your attention and not get hung up on the messy, difficult thoughts and feelings that may arise on the edges of your awareness.

PROACTIVELY ACCEPT YOUR LIMITATIONS IN DOING RELAXATION

In the practice of EPR, we treat ourselves as a loving mother treats her child, without judgment or impatience. If we get distracted easily, *if we are impatient or anxious, we practice being at ease with the intrusion of distraction while not succumbing to it.* If we cannot find patience, we rest with our impatience while focusing our attention. While we focus, we accept any discomfort that arises that pulls our attention away, every feeling, aversion, or unpleasantness that temporarily interrupts our focus. We practice accepting and resting, no matter how shallow and unsatisfying our relaxation might be, and remain steadfast in our focus on what is most relaxed within, however slight. We watch how distractible we are with kindness. We experiment being patient in noticing how our attention is diverted again and again by thoughts and feelings. We accept without judgment or impatience with all that briefly disturbs our peace in each moment.

NO THINKING

Paradoxical Relaxation *is a practice of not getting stuck in any thought, no matter how compelling.*

If a thought that feels important arises, we can write it down so as to get it out of our head. Other than that, when a thought arises, without analyzing it or thinking about it further, we practice taking our attention away from the thought and refocus on the *feeling* of relaxation. We allow ourselves to adopt the attitude "I don't have to think about anything right now."

We practice not being disturbed by how often we get caught in thinking, even if thoughts distract us every other second. Doing this repetitively improves with practice. We simply take our attention away from the distracting thought again and again, and rest in the sensation of what is most relaxed inside. Nothing in our awareness is to be judged or refused.

The twelfth-century poet Rumi said it eloquently:

Each of us is a bed-and-breakfast inn
Each day a new guest arrives at the door
A feeling of happiness, grief or heartbreak shows up
A sense of emptiness or love
Invite them all in and offer them tea
Even if your visitors seem ungrateful for your hospitality
And appear to want to ransack your lovely place
And steal everything, extend your hand
A distressing thought, unyielding tension, or feeling of
    dread
Greet each with good cheer
For each has come to help you on your way

> *Your attitude toward what is going on*
> *inside makes the difference between*
> *being able to deeply relax and not.*

In EPR you practice accepting the limitations and imperfections of your ability to let go, stay focused, and accept whatever arises. In doing this repetitively during your practice of relaxation, you'll grow more and more skilled at accepting and releasing yourself from your minor, usually unspoken, aversions. When you sit or lie down to do EPR, you direct your attention away from the outside world and into yourself, into your inner experience and inner life. There is a collage of experience inside your body and mind. If you're peaceful and happy, the experience is very pleasant: happy reveries, deep relaxation, and feelings of wholeness, lightness, and peace fill your body and mind.

> *It all happens in the now: you'll accept*
> *whatever is arising and falling away within you*
> *during relaxation, one moment at a time.*

When you're in pain or in a state of anxiety, depression, and irritation, in which you cannot see a positive future for yourself, your attention is drawn to all that fearfulness, which typically involves a nonstop stream of negative images that comprise a picture of your life in the moment that feels very bad.

Bringing your attention inside when there are feelings of emotional disturbance and/or physical pain is the last thing someone normally wants to do, because at first there appears to be no benefit in doing so. While I am not suggesting focusing on what is distressing, if there is any experience of what is distressing, we practice allowing it to be present somewhere in our awareness. When beginning EPR, there can be a stream of scary thoughts and feelings as you direct your attention inside, but it is still possible to focus in the midst of what may feel unpleasant or scary. When we practice EPR, sensation—subtle and often ignored when you're not feeling comfortable inside—is consciously brought into the foreground. If we have never practiced doing something like this, it can feel bewildering, strange, unwieldy, or impossible. When we finally understand the place we existentially stand in the adoption of the attitude I am describing above, it's easy and clear. The only way to find that out is by doing the practice over and over again. Ultimately we learn by repetitively practicing what we want to learn.

WHAT PROFOUND RELAXATION FEELS LIKE

Extended Paradoxical Relaxation is the practice of entering a sanctuary undisturbed by the world. Imagine during your day of emails, phone calls, bad news on TV—everything that Zorba the Greek called "the catastrophe of our life"—you could say, "Excuse me, I need to spend some time in heaven." Imagine you could walk through a door, close it behind you, and in a half an hour, you find yourself in paradise. Imagine, in the middle of your day, bringing yourself into a state where there's nothing to do, nowhere to go, no one to be, and nothing to accomplish. In this place, there's no fear; in this place, you carry no burdens and you feel at peace. Imagine practicing a method that can quiet your body, reduce or stop your pain, and allow the sore tissues of your pelvis to heal. *Extended Paradoxical Relaxation* is the practice of entering into this heaven-like refuge. This sanctuary isn't exactly how the movies might represent it or how Michelangelo painted it—no feasting rooms, seraphim, trumpets, angels, or pearly gates. There are no buildings, or mountains or streams; in fact, there are no forms at all, just a kind of weightless, joyful, floating feeling.

> *This inner haven that EPR helps you enter is open to those who have developed the ability to enter it.*

It is everyone's birthright—it comes with being born. When we see a baby sleeping or happily absorbed in playing with their mother, the baby is in this sanctuary.

> *Old mental habits, deeply ingrained in us from childhood, routinely keep us from being able to escape the stresses of the world and calm down inside.*

It can come to us momentarily as we're drifting off to sleep, in a moment of touching someone we love, during a massage, laughing with a child, or listening to beautiful music. This sanctuary is present in all of us all of the time, and we find it in the state of deepest relaxation, when our thinking stops.

> *For those who want it enough, these old habits can be overcome. With the kind of devoted practice of what I call* Extended Paradoxical Relaxation, *it is possible to overcome these habits and relax deeply almost any time you want to.*

WHAT HAPPENS WHEN YOU BECOME PROFOUNDLY RELAXED?

The term *bliss* is not too strong to describe the experience of profound relaxation. No anxiety, no worry exists in this state. No thought of future or past. The present moment is enough and is everything.

*Entrance into heaven comes to all who can
rest their attention outside of thinking.*

While some who become profoundly relaxed experience floating and weightlessness, others experience a feeling of heaviness, warmth, and tingling. Some have reported having a sense that they couldn't move, though there was no anxiety connected to this. Sometimes people in the moment of profound relaxation cannot determine whether they're lying on their back or on their stomach. When you become quiet during *Extended Paradoxical Relaxation,* as in other methods of quieting body and mind, you may experience a feeling of floating weightlessly.

As your tension decreases, you begin to feel yourself letting go of a kind of protective or defensive holding-on that you did not realize you'd been doing. In the depths of this relaxation, there's often a sense of coming home—of returning to a place of utter comfort that you've always known and that is as intimate to you as your breath.

*It is common during deep relaxation to experience
the sense of a weight being lifted from you.*

As you get into deeper states of relaxation, particularly states that go past the normal range of nervous system quieting you're familiar with, several unusual kinds of sensations and phenomena can occur. Sometimes episodic jerking is accompanied by a feeling of falling. The jerking is sometimes a kind of defensive reflex response to the sense of falling. At other times deeper levels of relaxation are accompanied by feelings of heaviness of the limbs and a tingling in the arms, hands, and feet. Sometimes, you might momentarily have the feeling that you cannot move (although you always can). Sometimes there's a sense of the body simply disappearing. Again, these are all characteristic of deeper states of relaxation.

Some people who have followed the relaxation protocol have had these experiences and were alarmed by them. In truth, however, such experiences tend to be good news, signposts on the road to training the body to forgo its habitual vigilant contraction and learn to relax.

Becoming competent in *Extended Paradoxical Relaxation* does not occur overnight.

> *When you practice EPR, you will repeatedly confront a multitude of obstacles that interfere with your ability to voluntarily relax anxiety and calm your nervous system. It is in allowing these obstacles again and again that you learn to overcome them.*

PROFOUND RELAXATION OFFERS RELIEF FROM ANXIETY

One simple way to describe EPR is that it is a way to release the grip of anxiety and the knot in the pelvis. This is a slow process, but generally the more you practice this method, the better you get at it. Stress, fear, worry, anxiety, and agitation are just different names for the same thing. The survival response of fear prompts us to fight, flee, or freeze.

The purpose of fear is usually to motivate us to run away from or fight what we feel is threatening. Fear feels bad. None of us likes to feel afraid or stressed. We all yearn for the feeling of peace and relaxation inside. It has been my experience that in the absence of fear there are the feelings of love, peace, and gratitude.

> *The inner experience of heaven exists in the absence of fear, anger, and emotional agitation.*

At first people do *Extended Paradoxical Relaxation* imperfectly and poorly, and people will frequently become frustrated with how difficult it is to focus their attention. Often, at the beginning it feels like you're getting nowhere. And only those who persevere find the quiet universe that resides in the core of just being—the great sanctuary . . . peaceful, unassailable, joyful, blissful, effulgent. And in the treatment of pelvic floor dysfunction, this perseverance can open the door to the healing of a chronically sore pelvic floor.

When you are constantly anxious, your nervous system is aroused, preventing you from being able to truly rest or relax. *Rest and relaxation are the body's medicine for the healing of sore pelvic tissue.* In my view, the inability to deeply relax over time paves the way for anxiety states and their related physical difficulties centrally including pelvic pain.

EXTENDED PARADOXICAL RELAXATION IS 1 PERCENT INSPIRATION AND 99 PERCENT PERSPIRATION

Thomas Edison reputedly said that genius is 1 percent inspiration and 99 percent perspiration. In EPR the inspiration is the instruction and the underlying concepts. The perspiration is the daily, persistent practice of the EPR itself.

When you are a novice learning relaxation, it is difficult to appreciate the centrality of one of the main instructions: allow the sensation of tension and anxiety to be present while focusing on what is able to relax. A novice more often than not *tries to relax* even though the instructions given in *Extended Paradoxical Relaxation* urge you to abandon exerting the effort of trying.

In EPR, you're specifically asked *not to try to relax* because you cannot try (i.e., use effort) to deeply relax (i.e., cease effort). After attempting this strategy again and again, beginners usually come to see that *trying to relax doesn't work.*

It is not uncommon for someone to do many sessions of relaxation before he or she is genuinely willing to experiment with these instructions; that is, willing to wholeheartedly allow tension and anxiety to be present without having to do anything about them while focusing attention on sensation. Each relaxation session is an experience of doing your best to get the practice right, even though it often feels like you've fallen short of the mark over and over. There is simply no way to succeed at EPR without facing the repeated experience of losing the focus of your attention. As a practitioner of this method, you must find your own way to persevere through these frustrations. The moment in which you're able to allow tension and anxiety to be present and not have to do anything about them is a defining moment. It can reverberate throughout your life as the stage is set for you to experiment with accepting what is.

The instructions of EPR to focus on what is able to relax within, serve to help you return to the proper focus and technique, moment to moment. It is easy to get lost in reactions of frustration, doubt, or a sense that nothing is happening. It is a central focus of this method to notice these reactions, to be a witness to being lost in frustration, and to refocus on the relaxation instructions without self-rebuke. It is natural to react negatively, however subtly, to straying from the instructions or becoming lost in thought or frustration. With an attitude of forgiveness and compassion for oneself, the idea is to simply come back into the focus of following the instructions. Even reacting negatively, though frustrating, should *simply be noticed without judgment.*

In *Extended Paradoxical Relaxation* we practice accepting our tendency to hold on to vigilance, defensiveness, worries, and guarding ourselves as a way of ultimately releasing them. The word *surrender* comes from the French *surrendre,* meaning "to give up." *Extended Paradoxical Relaxation* is a practice of letting go of inward guarding and tensing, a practice of giving up the heavy weight of our daily worries.

Once you've done everything you're able to do about situations in life that worry you, continued worry is usually a hopeless attempt to control what you cannot control. Worry is a certain kind of thinking:

Worrisome thoughts focus on the past or future, and are the cornerstone of anxiety and tension. Beyond the positive effect of motivating you to do whatever you need to do about any given situation, further worry usually only creates suffering.

The irrational premise of compulsive worrying
is that it is not safe for you to take your
attention off what you fear might happen.

In doing EPR, you practice shifting your attention away from all thoughts, including worrisome or happy thoughts. When you're tense or anxious, your attention is almost always focused in the future or the past. The practice of continually bringing your focus into the present moment of sensation places you upstream from the anxieties of past and future.

When your attention is taken away from
worrisome thinking, anxiety and tension
connected to worrisome thinking can cease.

The simple truth is that after you've done everything you can do about any situation, whatever is going to happen is going to happen. In my own life, over and over, I noticed an inner programming that did not allow me to take my attention off what was worrisome, even though I had no control over it. During a relaxation session, I make a decision to trust that it is safe for me to take my attention off worry. This decision and my ongoing practice have been vital in honing my ability to calm myself.

When you practice Extended Paradoxical
Relaxation *and rest your attention in sensation,*
you're thrust into the present moment where
worry about past and future doesn't enter.

MOTIVATION AND FINDING THE COURAGE TO DO EPR

Extended Paradoxical Relaxation offers a method to move past the real-life, moment-to-moment inner obstacles to just sit or lie down to do a relaxation session and calm down the nervous system. I designed the practice to help anyone who is anxious or in pain to help manage often-overwhelming distractions in order to enter into a state of conscious effortlessness.

It takes courage to do EPR. To profoundly relax, you are asked to lie down, stay awake, rest your attention in sensation, and allow anxiety or discomfort to come and go in your awareness without doing anything to change them. Our aversion to these feelings and what to do with that aversion sidetrack many people's attempts to put an end to their anxious state through their own efforts.

> *When you're anxious or in pain, it can be hard,*
> *often scary and unpleasant, to lie down for a*
> *relaxation session, because it means being alone with*
> *your pain, anxiety, discomfort, and uncertainty.*

The instructions for *Extended Paradoxical Relaxation* specifically address what to do with the subtle psychological resistances to lying down with anxiety and discomfort. They address the issue of attention and how central it is to commit yourself to developing the "muscle" of attention, and they focus directly on how to rise above your reflexive aversion to pain and move toward the pleasure of profound relaxation.

When you're motivated to learn relaxation, you're often upset emotionally in some way. These feelings are usually unexpressed; they remain inside and are felt as a kind of pressure, constriction, or deadness. When unresolved, they are obstacles to your nervous system calming down. During relaxation, fear, sadness, grief, anger, and frustration are among the emotions that may arise.

When you're anxious or chronically tense,
some deep part of you, usually unspoken,
feels like you need to protect you.

Anxiety and chronic tension are states of self-defense. In a kind of unconscious reasoning, some part of your mind believes that tension and anxiety are helping you stay safe. I discuss this later as pleasure anxiety, catastrophic thinking, and the desire to avoid disappointment by rejecting the experience of feeling safe. And we address them with the aim of overcoming their influence or they remain obstacles to our relaxation.

Pleasure anxiety and the fear of feeling safe and
undefended are not just concepts. They occur in
real people whose suffering is real. They are the
engine that drives people to compulsive working and
workaholism, among other self-defeating practices.

EXTENDED PARADOXICAL RELAXATION IS THE PRACTICE OF UNDEFENDING YOURSELF

When people who are anxious or who suffer from the symptoms of anxiety begin PR, they usually feel fear about letting go. Sometimes people are uneasy about what they'll find inside, or afraid that they might lose control, or that something bad will happen if they let down. Beneath all the agitation of the nervous system is one of peace, which has been a fundamental understanding in wisdom traditions through-out history.

If tension is part of how you defend yourself,
Extended Paradoxical Relaxation is the
practice of letting go of defending yourself.

DEVELOPING YOUR OWN PRACTICE OF EPR

The instructions of *Extended Paradoxical Relaxation* need only be trusted up to the point where you feel the ultimate safety of resting in the state of deep relaxation. It is important that I say: "Underneath all your suffering, your tension, anxiety, and pain, lies serenity. You need only trust my words until you have the experience of this yourself. Then it is yours, and you don't have to rely on what I say anymore. It is safe for you to rest with anxiety, fear, sorrow, and uncertainty because just underneath these disturbing emotions is the ease you're looking for."

In EPR, the foundation of treatment is the understanding that relaxation occurs in a state of mental quiet. Anxiety is a disturbance of your natural state of tranquillity. You never lose the capacity to rest in a state without fear. Emotional disturbances merely obscure your natural anxiety-free state of inner quiet.

*To become skilled in EPR, it is necessary
to be committed to daily practice.
Without real earnestness, reliable ongoing
ability to relax is impossible.*

THE UP-REGULATED NERVOUS SYSTEM

The term *up-regulated nervous system* has come into use to describe a chronically aroused nervous system operating too fast and at too high an idle speed. The up-regulated nervous system is like the engine of a car whose driver presses down on the gas pedal while in neutral. When the engine goes too fast for too long a time, the different parts of the car—like the drive shaft, fuel system, tires, and brakes—can be stressed to the point of dysfunction or failure.

Skillful practice of Extended Paradoxical Relaxation *allows you to regularly turn down your idle speed and lower your baseline level of anxiety.*

Words that describe an up-regulated nervous system include: *nervous, worried, in an anxiety state, sympathetically aroused, afraid, panicked.* Words that describe a down-regulated nervous system: *relaxed, peaceful, happy, harmonious, cool, calm.* Using the car engine analogy, the purpose of *Extended Paradoxical Relaxation* is to allow you to lift the hood, get into the engine, and properly adjust the lever that regulates how hard the engine works. By adjusting this lever, the engine can slow down to a normal speed that doesn't stress the engine or the parts of the car that it runs.

In his experiments at Harvard during the first part of the twentieth century, Walter Cannon, a doctor of physiology, professor and chairman of the Department of Physiology at Harvard Medical School (1871 to 1945), opened up the abdomen of a cat and noticed that the cat's bowel moved rhythmically and regularly, but when a dog was brought into the room, the peristaltic movement of the bowel stopped. In the first case, the cat was in a related parasympathetic state in which its bowel was purring. Enter a dog, and the rhythmic movement of the bowel stopped. When the dog was taken out of the room, the cat's bowel resumed peristalsis.

BRAIN ACTIVITY AND ATTENTION TRAINING

When you look at the hands of a carpenter, hands that are used to holding hammers, saws, and lumber, you notice that they're large and brawny. When you look at a ballerina who practices leaping and dancing *en pointe* every day, you see legs that are strong and muscular. Your body and mind develop to support any activity that you do repetitively. Whatever you practice, your body and mind will develop as a central part of being more skilled at what you are practicing.

The field of neuroscience has recently documented dramatic changes in the brain associated with repetitive activity. For instance, the part of the brain associated with the muscular activity of the fingers of the left hands of violinists shows dramatically more blood flow than the part of the brain associated with the activity of the fingers of the right hand, which simply holds the bow and isn't involved in the gymnastics of the fingers of the left hand.

A soldier held captive during the Korean War practiced golf in his mind while confined to a cell for a number of years. Every day, morning to evening, he would imagine every aspect of playing: gripping the club, planting his feet, each swing, long drives down the fairway, and short putts on the green. Remarkably, when he was freed and returned home, he was reputed to have scored under 100 in his very first game after having not physically touched a golf club for years. He had put in the necessary hours of "practice," but in his case the practice was in visualizing the game rather than actually playing it. This is a striking example of using controlled attention to visualize the honing of a skill that you would think could only be practiced on the golf course.

The golfer's story is consistent with recent discoveries about neuroplasticity, which have documented development of the brain through simple mental rehearsal of an activity. It appears you can practice playing the piano without even touching it, and you'll still strengthen the brain activity associated with playing.

Mastering any skill means practicing it repetitively.

What is remarkable in the emerging research is that paying attention is a specific kind of brain state that involves activation in parts of the brain that typically don't operate at the same time. Further, people who've practiced focusing their attention for thousands of hours demonstrate a level of brain activity associated with attention that is not seen in the brains of those who have not practiced attention training.

By the time I met my teacher, Edmund Jacobson, I calculate that he'd been practicing relaxation for approximately 25,000 hours. It has been said that musicians, tennis players, baseball pitchers, airplane pilots, machinists, and painters become masters of their art after they've put in 10,000 hours of practice. This means three hours of practice every day for ten years. The point is that just like a carpenter who must have strong hands to wield a hammer all day—and has to have developed increased brain activity to support accurate hammering—so the brain develops to support the activity of sustained attention.

> *The goal in* Extended Paradoxical Relaxation
> *is to maintain seamless, continuous,*
> *unbroken attention—no matter what your*
> *experience is during the relaxation.*

To grow competent in focusing attention requires many hours of practice to develop the brain activity associated with it. In other words, whether you're relaxing or not, whether you feel like you're getting anywhere or not, whether you feel happy or sad or good or bad, the goal in EPR is to maintain unwavering attention on what you are focusing, without trying to make anything release. In people with chronic anxiety, the nervous system and brain are used to being in an aroused state. If you tend to be anxious, you're good at practicing being anxious. Overcoming the tendency to live with an aroused nervous system means practicing what reduces this arousal.

Extended Paradoxical Relaxation doesn't work if you are lazy. It works best if you sincerely give yourself to carrying out its instructions. It works if you're willing to persevere through the myriad times you don't do the instructions perfectly. It works if you commit to unconditionally accepting yourself as you work with the instructions. It works if you're willing, on a moment-to-moment basis if necessary, to reassert your will to accept tension and anxiety and all that the practice entails. The continual assertion of your will refers to making a choice to keep your attention focused in a certain way.

REPEATED PRACTICE OF BEING UNCONDITIONAL WITH YOURSELF

When you direct your attention inside for extended periods, many emotions and reactions can arise in response to inner discomfort or anxiety. Your attitude toward these can facilitate or interfere with your relaxation. One major lesson for those dealing with anxiety is to learn to be unconditional with themselves regardless of what arises. By *unconditional,* I'm referring to an attitude of "I'm going to be present with myself whatever I experience inside. Whether I'm able to focus well or am distracted, whether my symptoms reduce in this moment or not, whether I'm able to accept my tension or not, I will be here for myself without limitations or conditions. I'll do whatever it takes, for as long as it takes, to help myself."

We usually treat ourselves the way our parents treated us. Few people have ideal childhoods in which their parents have the time, energy, emotional balance, and wisdom to love us unconditionally. We all want unconditional love, but few ever experience it beyond the fleeting moments of infancy. To be unconditional with yourself is to treat yourself the way you always wanted your parents to treat you.

Few of us have ever completely devoted ourselves to our own care. The relaxation protocol I'm describing requires time and patience. I often tell my patients that while there are some general parameters for how long it takes for their symptoms to abate, for *Extended Paradoxical Relaxation* to work it will take as long as it takes. The people who practice relaxation with this unconditional attitude seem to do the best.

The instruction to keep attention focused on sensation, especially for those who've had little experience with introspection, isn't easy at first, though it gets easier with practice.

For many, the world inside the body and mind is uncharted territory. Making subtle distinctions about their internal sensations is often difficult for my patients because it is an activity they haven't practiced. The inclination to avoid bringing attention inside the body is often, though not always, related to emotional pain that someone has simply wanted to escape from. If there are areas of discomfort in your body, there's a natural tendency to draw away from them. This often occurs when there's anxiety-related constriction or discomfort or some anxiety-related disorder. Your attention wants to focus anywhere but near the discomfort. We're all programmed to pursue pleasure and avoid pain, but successful practice of EPR requires that you direct your attention back into your body even if it is initially uncomfortable and that you do so with unconditional support of yourself.

> *How you come back from distraction is as*
> *important as maintaining sustained focus.*

When people first begin *Extended Paradoxical Relaxation* training, almost all of them report that their major frustration is staying focused. Their distress over being so often distracted by thoughts is usually allayed when they understand that the practice of EPR involves getting good at "coming back" from distraction, *which is as important as maintaining seamless focus.*

What defeats many people who want to learn relaxation is that they don't know what to do with what doesn't feel good inside during the session. Developing the ability to control your attention and cultivate undistracted focus is no different from the development of any other skill. Whether you want to learn to play the guitar, excel at tennis, or use a new computer language, it is a challenge to stay focused on what you've just begun to learn because you're asked to stay present with what feels uncomfortable and what you don't yet do well.

As an analogy, a good driver seamlessly and effortlessly makes these corrections without remorse or shame or reactivity. These corrections are done without a thought that you're doing anything other than driving well. When good drivers occasionally veer over the lane line, they don't consider it a bad thing or judge themselves negatively; it is just one of the things that happen when you drive.

*Being able to remorselessly return your
attention from distraction is a variation
on the practice of self-forgiveness.*

Being remorseless, shameless, and self-forgiving in doing *Extended Paradoxical Relaxation* will be deeply tied in with your ability to be self-forgiving about the mistakes you make in life. Self-forgiveness in the face of your errors is no small issue, and it is one of the benefits of PR: practicing self-forgiveness during relaxation helps you to practice it in your life.

*When we forgive ourselves is when we're
most likely to forgive others. When we're
unforgiving of ourselves, we treat others
similarly. The importance of shamelessness,
self-forgiveness, and remorselessness during
EPR cannot be emphasized enough.*

When you take the practice of being shameless, remorseless, and self-forgiving seriously with regard to losing focus when you're doing EPR, you become able to calm down in situations where you never thought it would be possible to relax, such as during an emotional upset with someone, a health crisis, or a delicate negotiation.

ATTENTION ON SENSATION VS. ATTENTION IN THINKING

How can you tell the difference between paying attention to sensation and paying attention to thinking? When you rest your attention in a neutral sensation, your mind and body tend to quiet down. You have to be in the present, neither going back to the past nor considering the future. Thoughts may flit in and out, but your attention rests on the sensations you feel. When your attention shifts to thinking, some increase in tension and discomfort usually occurs.

Just go to the center of the room, and put one chair in the center. Take the one seat in the center of the room, open the doors and windows, and see who comes to visit. You will witness all kinds of scenes and actors, all kinds of temptations and stories, everything imaginable. Your only job is to stay in your seat. You will see it arise and pass, and out of this, wisdom and understanding will come.

Ajahn Chah

You can teach somebody how to do a job, but only time makes them better. The longer they do it, the better they get at it.

Craftsman at Steinway piano factory

In contemporary parlance, practice simply means to do something over and over again. This applies whether you practice *Extended Paradoxical Relaxation* or craft the cabinets for concert pianos.

As a rule, you get better at whatever you practice. In my relaxation practice, I've discovered that if I don't stay on top of the tendency for my attention to waver, the quality of my relaxation suffers. If I miss doing relaxation for a day, my life suffers—simple as that.

In our pelvic pain clinics, we give our patients a sixty-lesson course that they need to do consistently over a long period of time once they leave the clinic. Regular daily practice is what makes it effective. This is essential for anyone who wants to use PR to reduce anxiety. When you get good at EPR, you can often regularly release yourself from pain and anxiety.

THERE'S NO SUBSTITUTE FOR PRACTICE

There are three rules to learning *Extended Paradoxical Relaxation*: Practice, practice, practice. The only way I've been able to improve my ability to quiet my body and mind is to practice controlling my attention, accepting whatever sensation I'm focused on, letting go of my preferences, and releasing my aversion to my fearful thoughts. Relaxation requires that I practice not resisting what is uncomfortable or painful, practice not arguing with reality, practice accepting and resting with whatever the sensation is, and practice letting go of the outcome.

IT IS HARD TO DIG THE WELL WHEN THE HOUSE IS ON FIRE

It is best to have dug a well before you desperately need the water. The image of digging the well when the house is already aflame illustrates the importance of preparation. In dealing with the crisis of my brother's illness and death, which made calming my highly agitated nervous system so difficult, I depended on the relaxation practice I had done when there was no crisis in my life. I had dug a rudimentary well in advance of the fire.

Having a practice to calm nervous arousal and enter into a tranquil state is especially important as you face the inevitable difficulties of aging or suffer the physical symptoms of anxiety-related disorders. Recently, I spoke to a friend whose eighteen-year-old son was leaving home, which left my friend to deal with empty nest syndrome. She has been practicing meditation for many years and can quiet her mind and body with unusual skill. She told me that although her son's departure and her changing role as a mother had its moments of discomfort, her meditation practice returned her to a place of deep inner relaxation and happiness.

Put on your own oxygen mask first. To stop feeling guilty about how much time you spend taking care of yourself, you will need to forgive yourself for your condition. If the biggest gift you can offer others is to take care of yourself and bring peace into your life, then self-judgments about your suffering make no sense. When I realized that the best thing I could do for my loved ones was to take care of myself, I had to find a way to forgive myself for having pelvic pain. I knew that if I'd been given a choice about pelvic pain, I would never have chosen to have it. I learned to stop taking my condition personally, as if it were the punishment for some mistake I'd made or some unforgivable sin I'd committed.

PUT YOUR OWN OXYGEN MASK ON FIRST

There's a good reason why the airlines tell you to don your own oxygen mask before you put on your children's masks. If you're gasping for breath, you'll be far less effective in helping others, and your panic will spill over to those you're trying to help. I've often told my patients that the biggest gift you can give those who love you and depend on you is to take care of yourself and to get better.

Think of the gift it would have been for you
if your mother or father had devoted time
for themselves each day to self-care and had
emerged feeling happier, more peaceful, more
emotionally available, and more giving.

Few of us would have resented their taking that time. On the contrary, we'd have wanted them to take care of themselves and we'd have gladly given up that time to them.

Most of the people I've treated for pelvic pain have been very conscientious about fulfilling their obligations and taking care of those who depended on them, but the significant, sometimes disabling distress of their own anxiety and related disorders was a major obstacle. Typically, though, when they calmed their inner pain, taking care of others became easy and joyful. The main insight of *Extended Paradoxical Relaxation* is that the relaxation of all sensations, including tension that won't easily relax, involves the acceptance of these sensations. This is a compelling idea, though it sounds contradictory. "Accepting tension to relax it" is a broad subject, and being able to practice it as well as intellectually grasp it is crucial to deepening your EPR practice. When you accept tension or discomfort, you are, again, neither adding anything to, nor subtracting anything from, the discomfort. You are simply lying alongside the tension. You are not doing anything about it except being present and feeling it.

The form of poetry known as haiku demonstrates the pure intention to accept what is. Here are two examples:

The crisp autumn leaves
Rustle softly in the wind
And then blow away
Warm night, gentle breeze,
The smell of jasmine heavy
In the summer air

In these poems the poet simply reports his experience of what is before him. There's no embellishment, no judgment, no interpretation of what he perceives, no spin.

Choosing to be okay with your inner experience sends a powerful message to your nervous system. When you practice regarding your inner experience, whatever it is, as okay, you tell your nervous system to stop secreting adrenaline and the biochemicals that arouse fight, flight, and freeze. This is a practice of self-soothing, an attitudinal change that stops the internal wars that often go on against your inner experience.

The practice of being okay tells your nervous system there's no danger, nothing to tighten up against or be aroused about. Being okay with tension and everything else that has felt unsafe inside, when practiced repeatedly, erodes the grip of chronic arousal of your sympathetic nervous system.

HOW DOES IT WORK?

One of the essential instructions in EPR is to be okay with the sensation you've chosen to focus on, whether it's painful or pleasurable. How do you do that?

Being okay with sensation, especially if it contains tension, requires your willingness to tell yourself that something is okay and to want to believe it. It is a profoundly personal choice to be okay with something; no one can force you into it. This is especially true when your first impulse is to not be okay with the sensation you're focusing on or the anxiety you feel.

When you accept whatever sensation is inside you, you simply feel it and make a moment-to-moment choice to do nothing about it. Resolving tension that you *can* control easily is a no-brainer. For example, when you tense your arm and can then relax it easily, there's no need to work with it because it dissolves by virtue of the easy instruction you give yourself. In contrast, the sensations that appear outside your control, that are often unpleasant, that won't relax readily no matter how strong or subtle, bring on the tension that you have to work with and accept. In accepting this residual tension and the discomfort it causes, we are also letting go of the desire in this moment *to be more relaxed and to feel more at ease or more whole.*

Accepting all sensations within you, including tensions or discomforts that persist in the moment, is like holding a baby—you keep your arms firmly on the baby while allowing it room to wiggle, move, or change position. Similarly, you focus your attention on the tension yet allow the sensation to move or change, which it will usually do again and again. Letting the tension or other sensation shift and squirm as you simply note it and accept it is important in the successful practice of EPR.

DEALING WITH THE TYRANNICAL CARETAKER

Extended Paradoxical Relaxation training is all about resting with *what is.* It is easy to relax a tightened fist: You tighten the muscles and then they relax easily when you decide to let go. What is outside most people's ability is to voluntarily relax contracted muscles and an aroused nervous system that don't respond to the wish to relax them. Resistance is what we call your body's refusal to relax. This refusal is primitive; it is on the level of a two-year-old shouting "NO!" Similarly, you cannot force an aroused nervous system to relax. Resistance to letting go is a defense against relaxation. There's no way to cheat this defense. It is unlikely that hypnosis and therapeutic suggestion, for example, or medication, surgery, or any other intervention that works from outside to inside, will bypass this conditioned resistance for long.

Most of us forget how emotionally open and vulnerable we were as children, how deeply life affected us on a moment-to-moment basis. We forget our intense grief at the thought of being abandoned when our parents left the room and were out of our sight. We forget that we did not understand the idea of the future, because we were forever living in the moment. We forget the terror and devastation of a parent's anger with us. When we hear the heartrending cry of an infant pulling us to comfort it, we forget that we used to be that infant.

> *As adults we forget the state we were in as young*
> *children when we had no shield against the*
> *tornado of our own emotions or those of others.*

When those emotions were positive, we could experience the joyful love and peace described in fairy tales. When those emotions were negative or threatening, we could feel a terror that made us feel like we were on the verge of annihilation.

The recall of this childhood universe can help clarify the stubbornness of the resistances to relaxation we experience in practicing *Extended Paradoxical Relaxation.* Clinical psychologist Donald Kalsched's exploration of early childhood trauma is instructive. *When the infant or young child is faced with what we now call abuse or trauma,* as Kalsched discusses in *The Inner World of Trauma,* a primitive, *a self-protective, reaction occurs to protect the overwhelmed child.* Kalsched variously names this reaction a protector/persecutor, or a tyrannical caretaker. He suggests that this reaction that occurs within a traumatized child is indeed the reaction of a tyrannical caretaker whose mission is self-protective but eventually misguided and self-destructive. He writes:

This primitive (tyrannical, caretaking) defense does not learn anything about realistic danger as the child grows up. It functions on the magical level of consciousness with the same level of awareness it had when the original trauma or traumas occurred. Each new life opportunity (to open, grow, and love) is mistakenly seen as a dangerous threat of retraumatization and is therefore attacked. . . .

Kalsched goes on to describe the ferocity
of this inner reaction in its single-minded
intention to protect whatever vestige of trust
in life may have survived the trauma.

He describes this peculiar self-destructive tendency of the psyche, to prevent even the possibility of further trauma by banishing all inner vulnerability, to being surprised by the kind of pain the individual has experienced. This explains the behavior of people who seem to sabotage every relationship they enter into: the protective reaction cannot allow them to open to the possibility of being hurt. Kalsched writes:

"Never again" says our tyrannical caretaker, "will the traumatized personal spirit of (my inner) child suffer this badly! Never again will (I) be this helpless in the face of cruel reality . . . before this happens I will disperse into fragments (dissociation) or encapsulate it and soothe it with fantasy (schizoid withdrawal) or numb it with intoxicating substances (addiction) or persecute it to keep it from hoping for life in this world (depression) . . . in this way I will preserve what is left of this permanently amputated childhood—of an innocence that has suffered too much too soon."

"If I forbid myself to be vulnerable
and unafraid, I'm safe."

When the inner experience of a young child is too painful for the child to process, a self-protective reaction forms as a defense. I characterized this psychic inner strategy when I described pleasure anxiety.

*The tyrannical caretaker says it is better to
remain closed to intimacy and dependency
than risk being vulnerable and suffer whatever
assault might occur in an unprotected state.*

Kalsched characterizes the different ways that a person defends against vulnerability and openness after unresolved trauma by using categories of dissociation, schizoid withdrawal, addiction, and depression. In fact, the defense isn't confined to these categories. What is called an earworm, a tune that goes around and around in your head, can also be considered obsessive thinking and may perform the same function of defending against feeling vulnerable. What Kalsched calls the tyrannical caretaker can be labeled a subpersonality, a defensive reaction, a splinter from the psyche, an enduring characterological posttraumatic stress disorder, or simply a defensive resistance to deep relaxation. The tyrant happens to be expressed physically in what I call the default inner posture, and psychologically in what I call pleasure anxiety.

*The resistance to fully relaxing, which
Jacobson called residual tension, when
given words, more often than not, turns
out to be the tyrannical caretaker.*

The default inner posture, pleasure anxiety, the tyrannical caretaker, a psychic splinter or subpersonality, and characterological posttraumatic stress disorder all sing the same tune. These terms are all descriptions, from different vantage points, of the same inner phenomenon. The script reads:

"If I feel safe, unafraid, spontaneous, unguarded, I'm in danger. I won't allow myself to be exposed and vulnerable to being surprised at being hurt. I might be hurt or rejected, but I won't be surprised by it."

The tyrannical caretaker defense doesn't arise only in people who've been traumatized; individuals who never experience trauma, who simply deal with the garden-variety suffering of childhood, can develop this same fierce inner defense.

In fact, this inner script of the tyrannical caretaker
occurs in people who haven't been abused
just as in those who have, and the defense
against deep relaxation in the non-abused
person can be just as fierce as in the abused.

The lie of the tyrannical caretaker is that remaining closed off, vigilant, and anxious will protect you from bad things.

The strategy of Extended Paradoxical Relaxation
is to bring into awareness and become friends
again with the part of us that refuses to relax.

WHAT LIFE IS LIKE WHEN RUN BY THE TYRANNICAL CARETAKER

The tyrannical caretaker doesn't want to hear that it cannot stop the blows of life. It is not interested in facts. It is a kind of hysterical, unreasoning clamping down to gain control over what cannot be controlled. It trades joy, spontaneity, love, openness, and peace for a bogus sense of security, in return for which it demands that you remain eternally afraid. It promotes the idea that you can be safe by always being aware that you're never safe. It tries to guard against what it cannot prevent by demanding that you live a miserable life of worry.

Yet no matter how hard the caretaker defense forces you to tighten up, or how long it stops you from letting go, it ultimately has no control over the whims of fate. If anything, in causing you to be chronically tensed, the tyrant promotes less competent judgment and ability to act. It distracts your attention from what you're doing. It keeps your nervous system in a fight-flight-freeze mode. Eventually it can compromise your immune system, can make you less attractive to others because of your joylessness and anxiety, and most important, it can rob you of your inner peace. Most people never examine or challenge their tyrannical caretaker in them. In EPR, we face it.

The tyrannical caretaker defense is typically unconscious. When this tension is given words, as I ask patients to give their residual tension words when I help them identify their default inner posture, the purpose of the tension makes no sense. Often, when people get in touch with it and learn about it, they're stunned.

The tyrannical caretaker defense is harsh, unyielding, and irrational. If bad things happen, it wants us to be prepared. It is a primitive reaction, unmoved by what by any standard is reasonable, loving, and good. Asked if there is ever a moment when it is okay to completely let go and be unguarded, the inner resistance says, "Never." Fun is not in its vocabulary. It is all business—in the service of survival, of protecting you by being on guard and not surprised by pain or danger. It refuses to accept the inherent transience and uncertainty of life. For this defensive reaction, the end of not being surprised by bad things justifies the means of inflicting fear and pain on oneself if that is what it takes.

Indeed, the tyrannical caretaker is not a thing,
not a demon inhabiting us. It is simply a primitive
dysfunctional reaction that we must not go to
war against if we want to become free of it. If
we try to combat the tyrannical caretaker or any
other unconscious inner reaction, we harden it.

EXTENDED PARADOXICAL RELAXATION IS PRACTICING LOVING-KINDNESS TOWARD ONESELF

When you view resistance to relaxation as the body's attempt to remain guarded in the illusory face of danger, the strategy of EPR becomes clear: In EPR, we face the tyrannical caretaker with loving-kindness. This is the only effective way to deal with this distressing and debilitating primitive reaction.

In Extended Paradoxical Relaxation, *we*
practice behaving toward our resistance
as a kind, loving, and patient parent.

We bring continuous unconditional attention to the part of us that is fearful, guarded, and not amenable to reason. We offer loving-kindness to a part of us that is closed off to life, love, openness, joy, and freedom. We make no demands on this part of us. We don't force or cajole or try to push it beyond what it is comfortable with in the moment. But we also don't allow the tyrannical caretaker to hold our attention captive. In EPR, we assert our will by resting our attention in sensation despite the protests of this part of us that doesn't want attention taken away from worrisome thoughts.

It is with the strategy of profound, focused attention, giving up all attachment to an outcome, that this terrified and resistant part of us can lay down its hopeless mission and let us open our hearts, to let go of defending against our experience of being and allow us to release our pelvic guarding.

FIGHTING THE REBEL IN YOU
ONLY SUPPORTS REBELLION

Continue the practice with the idea
that it is fine if you never relax.

A battle against the tyrannical caretaker will thwart our relaxation practice. Such confrontation consumes energy and keeps the nervous system aroused. The key to ending this battle with the part of us that doesn't want to cooperate with the relaxation instructions is to notice it and immediately accept it. What this means in practical terms is that *when you feel resistance to the subtle activity of accepting discomfort, simply feel this discomfort.* Most important, we make it okay that nothing has to happen. In allowing your resistance to accept the tension, you may become aware of feeling unpleasant sensations of restlessness or impatience. When you hear the instruction that says it is okay to feel these sensations, in wanting to do the method correctly, you notice any part of you that doesn't want to play along. If the rebellious part of you, which is wordless when it comes into your awareness, could speak, it would say, "I don't want to feel that." This physical resistance to feeling unpleasant sensations usually shows up as a kind of tension.

Permitting aversion and resistance to what you're averse to goes against our cultural orientation regarding what to do with pain. This instruction says your job during relaxation is not to take an aspirin, not to distract yourself, not to eat, drink, smoke, or do anything else to get away from the discomfort you're feeling. Instead, you turn toward the discomfort without attachment. You rest alongside the tension or discomfort and, on a moment-by-moment basis, renounce your urge to try to get anywhere or try to make the discomfort better. Paradoxically, this is the fastest way to release the tension and discomfort.

SAYING YES TO A LOUD INNER NO

In Extended Paradoxical Relaxation,
*we practice assuming an inner attitude
of saying yes to everything.*

We practice saying yes to the unconscious no inside us, which we seem to have little control over. *Extended Paradoxical Relaxation* is the practice of accepting everything in your experience as it is in the moment. This is the practice of nonresistance, nonclinging, nonattachment. Whatever is here in this moment is what we practice feeling and what we allow to exist without judgment or resistance. Doing this is the fastest way to calm nervous arousal.

In the musical *Fiddler on the Roof,* two men having a dispute bring their quarrel to the rabbi. One man says, "It was a horse." The other insists, "It was a mule." To the first man, the rabbi says, "You're right." Turning to the second man, the rabbi says, "You're right." A bystander asks the rabbi, "How can they both be right?" To this man the rabbi says, "You're right too." In *Extended Paradoxical Relaxation,* all of the constrictions, inner argument, discomforts, and resistances are right. Again, paradoxically, by honoring them all you facilitate their quickest resolution.

MOMENT-TO-MOMENT AND *EXTENDED PARADOXICAL RELAXATION*

The word *relax* comes from the old French word *relaxer,* which means "to make less compact or dense, to loosen, or open," and from the Latin word *laxus,* which means "to be wide, loose, open, slack, or languid." Indeed, tension is a state of denseness, tightness, constriction, and contraction. In the case of pelvic pain, relaxation aims to reverse a dense, tight, constricted, and contracted pelvic floor basin.

> Extended Paradoxical Relaxation *is the practice of conscious effortlessness.*

In our treatment protocol, we use *Extended Paradoxical Relaxation* in two different but complementary ways. Moment-to-moment *Extended Paradoxical Relaxation* is used throughout your normal day to regularly interrupt the habit of tensing the pelvic muscles. Doing moment-to-moment *Extended Paradoxical Relaxation* can involve many brief relaxations during the day. As you become more skilled, this practice takes less time and is done almost automatically. The intention here is for you to abort the old, dysfunctional chronic habit of tensing. *Extended Paradoxi-*

cal Relaxation requires setting aside time that is devoted to the practice of the technique, without the distractions that occur during your normal everyday life. This is best practiced two to three times a day, with each practice period lasting approximately thirty to forty-five minutes.

> *The skill of resting attention in sensation*
> *outside of thinking can make it possible for*
> *pain to reduce or disappear is developed in the*
> Extended Paradoxical Relaxation *practice.*

Moment-to-moment relaxation does not offer the depth of relaxation achieved by *Extended Paradoxical Relaxation*. By itself it has clear but limited effects. The intensive practice represents the laboratory in which the skill of relaxation is developed and represents the heart of the practice that produces the most benefit.

Moment-to-Moment Relaxation

Moment-to-moment relaxation is the practice of allowing the pelvic muscles to drop and relax at various moments throughout the day, whether you remind yourself spontaneously or use a reminding device. Under normal circumstances most people would rarely be willing to devote this kind of time and attention to change the habit of tightening up the pelvis either under stress or as a protective guarding response against pain felt in the pelvis. But most patients will devote the time and effort when they feel that doing so reduces their symptoms. Peculiarly, this motivation is the gift of this condition, even though it rarely feels like a gift when the symptoms exist unabated.

It is necessary to become aware of your habit of tensing the pelvic muscles on a moment-to-moment basis and change this habit. Throughout the day one checks for tension in the pelvic muscles to apply the technique of relaxing it. This is done many times, as long as these mini-relaxations don't interfere with normal functioning during the day. Sometimes one may want to tie a string around a finger, or paste a colored piece of paper to a bathroom mirror, or paste a tiny iridescent dot on a watch face. It is sometimes useful to use a small and inexpensive device called the MotivAider. Recently, certain vibration watches have come on the market that can be set to vibrate for certain set periods of time. These devices vibrate silently and repeatedly, like someone tapping you on the shoulder at times you designate, to remind you to let go of any tension unnecessarily being held in the pelvis. These devices can be set to vibrate every ten minutes, or every hour, as a private reminder to relax the pelvic muscles.

Sensing Pelvic Tension

Most people can feel tension in their pelvis and let go of this tension to some degree or another when they are aware of it. Others cannot. If you are one of those who cannot discern pelvic tension or how to relax pelvic tension, you can become sensitive to it in the following way. While you are sitting on a toilet, notice how your sphincter, rectum, and genitals slightly drop and relax when you begin to urinate. The sensation is very subtle and will occur out of awareness if you're not paying careful attention. These muscles naturally relax when you begin urination. These are the muscles that you want to learn to relax throughout the day, for these muscles are part of the guarding response that keeps the pelvic floor tight and tense.

Up Tight and Stuck Up

The relaxed, dropped state of the pelvic muscles tends to be absent with pelvic pain. Another way to conceive of what goes on in the pelvic floor is to understand that the tight and contracted pelvic muscles are stuck in a contraction and held up in such a contraction.

Don't look for immediate results. Don't strain in any way. It should just take a moment to notice and do and should hardly take any attention away from what you're involved in. Remember that your voluntary relaxation of these muscles at first will rarely cause much of a sense of relaxation in them. It is best to expect that your voluntary relaxation will only help a little to relax the pelvic muscles. Even if this method is effective for you, you may experience only slight relief of symptoms for days or weeks.

> *Moment-to-moment relaxation on an ongoing*
> *basis becomes a habit replacing the tendency*
> *to chronically tighten the pelvic floor.*

Hints on Doing Moment-to-Moment Relaxation

1. It Takes Time to Learn.

   It takes time to learn how to do moment-to-moment relaxation so that it does not interrupt your day. Doing it should take only a moment or two.

2. Make Sure That You Do Not Exert Effort.

   Make sure you do not exert any effort to relax. Just as you don't exert effort to initiate urination, don't exert effort to do this momentary relaxation. Don't push down as in the Valsalva maneuver, and don't do a Kegel exercise of tightening and then relaxing. Instead, just let go of any tension that you can easily let go of.

3. Continue to Practice Even If No Results Seem to Occur.

   Doing moment-to-moment relaxation is like using a thimble to empty water from a rowboat. Occasionally the effect on symptoms is dramatic; often it is not. *We tell our patients to continue to do it whether they have results or not.* Practicing this conscientiously for weeks has helped some patients reduce their symptoms.

> *The moment-to-moment relaxation practice*
> *is aimed at subtracting tension from the*
> *pelvic muscles throughout the day.*

Some people experience no benefit from doing this relaxation. On the other hand, in one unusual case, a man reported that doing this for several months reduced his symptoms by 90 percent.

RESPIRATORY SINUS ARRHYTHMIA BREATHING (RSA BREATHING)

RSA breathing is a description of the relationship between heart rate and breathing and refers to the heart rate varying in response to respiration. RSA is a phenomenon that occurs in all vertebrates. You can experience the phenomenon of RSA by taking your pulse and noting that when you breathe in, the heart rate increases slightly and when you breathe out the heart rate decreases slightly. Considerable research indicates that when there is balance and health, the heart rate and the breath move robustly together. In a normal healthy individual, as inhalation occurs, heart rate increases, and as exhalation occurs, heart rate drops.

Under circumstances of mental or physical disease, the relationship between breathing and heart rate is interrupted. When individuals suffer panic attacks, for instance, RSA is disturbed. When they recover from panic disorders their RSA breathing becomes more coordinated, stronger, more balanced, and robust. The higher, stronger, and more coordinated the heart rate is with respiration, the more balanced and healthy the individual. For example, healthy children generally have very robust RSA breathing in which the heart rate can sometimes vary forty beats or more between inhalation and exhalation.

It is usually possible with our RSA method to voluntarily strengthen RSA and bring it into balance. Restoring RSA can facilitate autonomic quieting and a reduction of anxiety by consciously coordinating the heart rate with respiration. We use this practice as part of paradoxical relaxation.

*Coordinating heartbeat and breath can help
calm down nervous system arousal.*

RSA-focused breathing should be done under the supervision of a professional. Occasionally, RSA can trigger benign ectopic or missed heartbeats. Light-headedness or a sense of not getting enough air can occur when it is not done correctly. If you find yourself feeling like that, take a break and try again. RSA can be a useful method to quickly quiet sympathetic nervous system arousal, reduce anxiety, and allow one to be at a deeper level of relaxation at the beginning of paradoxical relaxation.

Practicing RSA Breathing

It is generally agreed that slow, abdominal breathing in which the abdomen rises during inhalation and falls back during exhalation can be important in relaxation of the body and in the reduction of autonomic arousal. Slow abdominal breathing maximizes the possibility of breathing and heart rate coming into synchronicity with each other. While there is no absolute formula rigidly defining how many respirations per minute should occur to permit deep relaxation, six deep abdominal breaths per minute is considered more or less an optimal respiration rate. Breathing rates that accomplish preliminary quieting of the body can vary from two to nine breaths per minute depending on idiosyncrasies, experience, and metabolic requirements of the particular patient.

More important than having an idea of what the ideal number of breaths per minute should be is the understanding that one's level of comfort in breathing is the most important criterion in fine-tuning one's respiration rate during RSA breathing. When our patients slow their breathing to approximately six breaths per minute, as we will describe below, we ask them to adjust this slower respiration rate up or down to fit individual levels of comfort.

Computing the Number of Heartbeats Per Breath in RSA Breathing

In *Extended Paradoxical Relaxation,* RSA breathing can be done for approximately five minutes immediately prior to following the instruction for EPR. To determine how many heartbeats should be devoted to inhalation and how many heartbeats should be devoted to exhalation, we use the following computations (which may appear to make the technique more complicated than it is):

Patients are asked to take their pulse to determine their heart rate. Generally speaking, the heart rate is taken and monitored using the thumb of one hand to feel the pulse in the wrist of the other. Counting how many heartbeats occur in a fifteen-second time frame, and then multiplying that number by 4, is an easy way to determine the pulse rate per minute.

We ask patients to divide their heart rate by 6. If, for instance, someone has a heart rate of around 60 beats per minute the computation would be:

60 / 6 = 10 (Represents the number of beats allocated for a full
in and out breath in order to breathe six times per minute)

We then would divide 10 by 2 to get the number 5. Similarly, if someone has a heart rate of around 72 beats per minute, 72 divided by 6 equals 12, and 12 divided by 2 equals 6. The number 6 in this case or the number 5 in the previous case represents the number of heartbeats allocated for a single inhalation or exhalation.

Patients lie down in preparation to do EPR. We ask them to be in a comfortable position while feeling their pulse. Sometimes pillows are placed under the elbows to reduce the tension in the arms and hands while they feel the heart rate. This makes it easier to feel the pulse on an ongoing basis.

Once relaxed and feeling the pulse comfortably, patients with a heart rate of between 55 and 64 are instructed to inhale over a count of five heartbeats and exhale over a count of five heartbeats. Similarly, if the heart rate is between 65 and 74, six heartbeats are counted during inhalation and six heartbeats are counted during exhalation. If one's heart rate is between 75 and 84, seven heartbeats are counted during inhalation and seven heartbeats are counted during exhalation.

The amount of air taken in can vary. If patients feel that they are not getting enough air, they take in more air. If they feel uncomfortable getting too much air, they reduce the intake of air. Breathing in or out more can be done more quickly at the beginning, middle, or end of the appropriate heartbeat count, depending on what feels comfortable.

Breathing must be *comfortable*. Comfort level is the most important fact in considering whether to breathe in or out more or less, or whether to breathe more quickly or slowly at any given part of the breathing cycle. As in paradoxical relaxation, attention is returned over and over again back to the sensation of the breath, away from attending to visual or conceptual thinking. Usually after about five minutes, one begins EPR without regulating or paying attention to the breath at all.

RSA BREATHING AS A MEANS TO QUIET DOWN URINARY FREQUENCY AND URGENCY

Some patients have reported that the practice of RSA breathing has quieted down the urge to urinate. One of our patients who felt the urge to urinate was stuck on an airplane runway and had to remain seated for an hour. He did the RSA breathing and reported that he was nearly able to stop his sense of urinary urgency. We have had others who have reported that they have been able to use skin rolling (discussed later) to accomplish this as well.

RESTING ATTENTION IN SENSATION AND NOT IN THOUGHT

We all understand what it means to think what can be called a picture thought, a verbal thought, or an abstract thought. If you imagine an apple, what you're seeing in your mind's eye can be called a picture thought. When you think about what you said to a friend yesterday, your focus is on what can be called a verbal thought. When you add 420 to 816, your focus is on what can be called an abstract thought. Thoughts are symbolic representations in the mind.

Extended Paradoxical Relaxation
is the practice of not thinking.

Sensation can be felt directly without the need for thought. When you feel a cold wind on your face, your attention is directed to sensation directly. No thought is necessary.

*A central premise of EPR is that
relaxation occurs when attention rests
in sensation and not in thought.*

In fact, relaxation is most profound when no thought is absent. Learning EPR requires that you can make the distinction between a thought and a sensation and that you can rest attention in sensation.

It is essential to become practiced in focusing attention on sensation and not on a picture or thought of it. When you slip into a warm fragrant bath, you feel the warmth and support of the water and smell the fragrance in it. The bath experience is sensory and not intellectual.

*Streams of thought will typically arise in the
mind while you are doing* Extended Paradoxical
Relaxation. *Simply pay no attention to them
and continue to rest attention in sensation.*

However, correctly focusing on sensation in no way means that thoughts should not come into your awareness. Very often one can be absorbed in sensation while peripherally noticing thoughts coming in and out of awareness. This is absolutely fine. Becoming an adept in *Extended Paradoxical Relaxation* means that you can stay focused on sensation as thoughts float in and out of awareness and not have your attention be pulled away by these thoughts.

GETTING GOOD AT *COMING BACK*

Morihei Ueshiba, known as the father of the modern martial art of aikido, was reputedly asked by one of his students how he remained so present and apparently unperturbed in the midst of a fight. Whether the story is apocryphal or not, he is reputed to have said that he did not consider himself particularly good at being continuously present in a fight but that what he was really good at was "coming back" from being distracted.

When people first begin *Extended Paradoxical Relaxation* training, almost universally they report that their major difficulty is staying focused. Their distress about being distracted is usually allayed when they understand that the practice of *Extended Paradoxical Relaxation* involves, like the skill of the aikido master, getting good at "coming back" from distraction. One learns to be tireless, remorseless, and unperturbed by the tendency of one's mind to wander away from the object of focus.

Coming right back from distraction without emotion or internal comment is what it takes to get good at "coming back." There is no quick way to achieve this—practice, practice, and more practice is the secret.

SUBTLETIES IN THE PRACTICE

Engaging in the activity of quieting down your nervous system and relaxing your pelvic muscles is a peculiar activity, unlike any other. The skill needed to do this involves the subtle control of your attention. It involves the micromanagement of your emotions and attitude in the moment of practicing *Extended Paradoxical Relaxation*. Absent the development of these skills, *Extended Paradoxical Relaxation* fails. In this section we will discuss these subtleties.

When you rest attention in neutral sensation, your mind and body tend to quiet down. When you pay attention to sensation, you have to be in the present, neither going back to the past nor considering the future. Thoughts may flit in and out, but your attention rests on the sensations you are feeling. When attention shifts to thinking, some increase in tension and discomfort usually occurs.

During *Extended Paradoxical Relaxation*, when you pay attention to slight amounts of tension in a part of your body, you typically notice fleeting thoughts. It is best to continue your focus on this slight amount of tension, resolutely returning when you are distracted by these thoughts.

When you are walking down a crowded city sidewalk, many faces come toward you as they continue in the opposite direction. If you are clear about where you are going, you continue in your direction. While you may see many of the faces at the periphery of your vision, you don't stop to have conversations with these people. You simply go in your direction.

NOWHERE TO GO, NOTHING TO DO, NO GOAL TO ACHIEVE

In the moment of deep relaxation, you are going nowhere, doing nothing, and not trying to achieve anything.

While doing EPR, it is important to remain aware of the inclination to do something about the tension you are feeling. In the beginning of *Extended Paradoxical Relaxation* people sometimes report feeling restless, which may incline them to want to wiggle or move to relieve their sense of uneasiness in the tension. In the first few minutes of relaxation, we usually suggest that the patient allow this wiggling or movement. As the relaxation proceeds, this inclination to wiggle tends to diminish, and with practice the nervous system and the muscles tend to quiet down.

YOU GIVE IT UP TO GET IT

Our purpose for doing *Extended Paradoxical Relaxation* is to achieve profound relaxation of the pelvic muscles and a significant reduction of nervous system activity to enable the healing of the sore pelvic tissue. Understanding this principle of giving up attachment to relaxation while feeling and accepting whatever sensation remains after you have relaxed your tension as much as you can will allow you a level of relaxation not available otherwise.

IDENTIFYING THE THOUGHT "IF I AM NOT TENSE, I AM NOT SAFE"

The chronically tight pelvis tends to be part of the habit of conditioned vigilance—a vigilance that says, "Beyond a certain point it's not safe for me to relax and take my attention off the external world." It often is an expression of an early conditioning that says, "If I am not on my guard, I am in danger."

> *There is no way to sneak around the resistance to letting go of tension. The most likely way to relax the resistance is to acknowledge and accept it.*

So almost universally, individuals with pelvic pain who tend toward anxiety bump up against a stubborn barrier to quieting down, relaxing their muscle tension, and allowing their level of arousal and guardedness to release. It is common for individuals with pelvic pain to feel that if they take their attention off the pelvic pain they are somehow unsafe. This stubborn barrier to relaxation is not arbitrary. We believe it is most likely to have been conditioned early in life. It is often a scary experience to relax this barrier.

The inner refusal to fully let go is "resistance"—resistance that is defending against relaxation. Let us be clear that there is no way to cheat this defense. In our view, it is unlikely that hypnotizing someone and waving the magic wand of therapeutic suggestion, for example, or giving medication or doing surgery, or using other interventions that work from the outside to the inside, will bypass or short-circuit this conditioned resistance.

MORE ON KRIYAS, FASCICULATION, FLUTTERING, JERKING, FEELING OF FALLING, BODY HEAVINESS, LIMB TINGLING, AND FLOATING

As one gets into deeper states of relaxation, particularly states that go past the normal range of nervous system quiet that one is familiar with, several unusual kinds of sensations and phenomena can occur. One can experience a kind of jerking and temporary tightening and relaxation of certain muscle groups at certain stages of *Extended Paradoxical Relaxation*. These are due to a kind of psychophysical ambivalence of letting go of vigilance beyond a certain point. It is as if the body and mind were saying: "I am letting go now, but as I let go I am not comfortable letting go to the extent I find myself letting go . . . so I tighten back up to guard against letting go too much, then I let go and go past the point of comfortable letting go and so I tighten up again."

Sometimes episodic jerking is accompanied by a feeling of falling. The jerking is a defensive response to the sense of falling. At other times deeper levels of relaxation are accompanied by feelings of heaviness of the limbs and a tingling in the arms, hands, and feet. Sometimes, for a moment, one has the feeling that one cannot move (although one always can). Again, these are all characteristic of deeper states of relaxation.

The episodic jerking or fluttering that can occur in the pelvis or elsewhere during relaxation may be due to a kind of psychophysical ambivalence toward letting go of vigilance. These sensations often occur when someone's pelvic muscles begin to relax.

In yoga, these movements are called kriyas and are thought of as involuntary movements, the release of physical, mental, or emotional tension as the life force of kundalini moves through areas of tightness. Kriyas are thought to be cleansing and indicative of moving toward a more developed state of consciousness.

It is common, as a very tight pelvic floor begins to relax, for one to feel a kind of fluttering or fasciculation in the muscles of the pelvis. It is usually pleasant and is usually accompanied by a reduction or stopping of pelvic discomfort or pain. Again, this feeling represents a kind of pelvic ambivalence about letting go, as if the muscles of the pelvic floor can't decide whether to relax or tighten.

CONTROLLING THE NERVOUS SYSTEM BY CONTROLLING ATTENTION

At the beginning of the twentieth century when airplanes first came on the scene, the lever that controlled their movement and direction was named the *joystick*. Attention is the joystick of the nervous system.

If you are able to control your attention,
generally speaking, you will be able to exercise
significant control over your nervous system.

For example, if you direct your attention toward something upsetting, your nervous system will immediately respond with arousal and disturbance. If you direct your attention toward what is peaceful and uneventful, your nervous system will remain quiet. All things being equal, when you can control your attention, you most likely control whether your nervous system is quiet or not.

You can think of the human organism as a "response machine," adjusting and responding to the different circumstances in the environment in order to survive. A central function of the nervous system is to respond with arousal to danger, to fight/flee/freeze. When attention is not directed to anything fearful or disturbing, the parasympathetic branch of the autonomic nervous system is activated, and restorative activities of tissue rejuvenation, healing, and rest dominate your experience. On the other hand, if you pay attention only to what is threatening, scary, ugly, and disturbing, the sympathetic branch of your nervous system is aroused and activated.

The point in Extended Paradoxical Relaxation
is to rest attention in sensation and to turn
attention away from the thoughts and
interpretations that pass through awareness.

In *Extended Paradoxical Relaxation* we practice simply receiving sensation directly, bypassing any filter through which the sensation usually passes. Absent any attention to thought, the nervous system remains quiet; electrical activity in the trigger points of the pelvic pain patient becomes unremarkable, as demonstrated by the many experiments of Gevirtz and Hubbard; and a reduction of pelvic pain and discomfort in that moment is very likely. Controlling attention without strain is the key to the success of *Extended Paradoxical Relaxation.*

NOW, NOW, NOW, AND MORE NOW

Be present now. Feel the tension now. Rest with the tension now. Take your mind back from wandering now. Feel the tension without interfering with it now. Accept the tension now. These and other instructions in *Extended Paradoxical Relaxation* are intimately tied to the present. *Extended Paradoxical Relaxation* only works as your attention is here and now. Voluntary relaxation of the pelvic muscles almost always occurs when attention is focused in the present moment.

Profound relaxation that allows the
pelvic floor to deeply relax is always
experienced in the present moment.

The commitment to keeping attention in the present moment often flies against the ingrained habits of thought that carry us back and forth from the past to the future. Being in this present moment often requires that you experience the discomfort and dysfunction that are hallmarks of pelvic pain. *It is the commitment to keeping your attention in the present moment that can allow the voluntary undoing of the discomfort and dysfunction.* Disregarding thoughts of the future and being present now are requirements of effective practice. All of the instructions in *Extended Paradoxical Relaxation* are done *now*.

THE INTERNAL MAP OF THE PSYCHOPHYSICAL TERRITORY OF *EXTENDED PARADOXICAL RELAXATION*

To most patients, pelvic pain is a mysterious condition, complete with weird pain and symptoms that don't go away, often wax and wane, and sometimes move from one place in the body to another. The person with pelvic pain typically experiences pain and symptoms no one else in their circle of friends has ever had. Because pelvic pain symptoms can't be seen and can't be identified by any of the objective testing that is normally used in medicine, and whose nature is not intuitively clear, most doctors do not really understand these symptoms either.

What is abundantly clear, however, is that at the heart of pelvic pain disorders is the presence of sore and irritated tissue inside the pelvic floor, most noticeable in its exquisite pain and sensitivity to touch and palpation. In pelvic pain disorders, there are also painful areas related to pelvic floor pain outside the pelvic floor. In a word, painful trigger points and sore, irritated tissue inside and outside the pelvic floor is the rule with those complaining of pelvic pain. Examining physicians often do not know how to examine this tissue or what to make of it. Many of our patients report that doctors they have seen will often scratch their heads and tell them that there is nothing wrong with them. Sadly doctors will sometimes diagnose this problem as a psychiatric one, or offer drugs or procedures that don't help and sometimes complicate or exacerbate the problem.

Over the years, as we have been treating pelvic pain, we have come to understand it in a way that is missed by the larger group of those who treat pelvic pain. I happen to believe our concept is the closest concept to the reality of pelvic floor–related pain. It comes from a deep experience of pelvic pain and its resolution and from our group having had the advantage of treating thousands of patients over the years.

Simply put, our understanding is that pelvic floor dysfunction is a kind of irritated *charley horse* in the pelvic floor that is caught in a cycle of tissue irritability, spasm, reflex protective guarding, pain, and anxiety.

Our understanding of chronic pelvic pain syndromes is that anxiety-related chronic physical tightening in the pelvis over time, or a physical injury in or around the pelvis, can cause what is commonly regarded in conventional medicine as an unremarkable irritation of muscle tissue of the pelvic floor. This irritated pelvic floor tissue is at the mildest end of the spectrum of disturbance occurring to human tissue. It is not cancer, infection, fungus, inflammation, contusion, edema, or necrosis. It is reversible irritation caught in a web of psychophysical events that interfere with its healing. Nevertheless, *what is thought of as unremarkable irritation of the pelvic floor tissue is the heart of the miserable condition of pelvic floor dysfunction. When the tissue heals up and stops being sore and irritated, pain and dysfunction resolve.*

Earlier, we have proposed that pelvic floor tissue irritation and its related pain, brought about by chronic tightening, *triggers a reflex pelvic floor protective guarding.* In other words, the pelvic floor tissue has a protective reflex to tighten up when it is in pain, much as an amoeba reflexively contracts when you prick it with a needle. When pelvic tissue is sore or irritated, its reflex protective response is to tighten up and pull into itself.

This reflex pelvic protective muscle guarding is dysfunctional because it increases pain, reduces blood flow, and *increases* protective guarding against the pain. This is all part of a dysfunctional, self-feeding cycle that is triggered. All of this typically triggers anxiety and catastrophic thinking that the pelvic pain will never go away. Thus, we describe the *self-feeding cycle of anxiety-producing pelvic tension, leading to tissue irritation, reflex protective guarding, pain, and increased anxiety. This cycle takes on a life of its own and is the heart of the chronic part of chronic pelvic pain syndromes.*

BREAKING THE PELVIC PAIN SELF-FEEDING CYCLE AND *EXTENDED PARADOXICAL RELAXATION*

The *Wise-Anderson Protocol*'s purpose is to give patients tools to break this cycle, enabling the healing of the sore pelvic tissue and the cessation of pelvic floor tightening under stress. We consider it essential to teach our patients to release the chronic, tissue-irritating, and painful protective guarding *physically* through internal and external myofascial trigger point release. Then, critically, our protocol calls for the pelvic pain patient to create a daily environment for their irritated painful tissue to heal. This daily environment means that the pelvic pain patient learns to physically release the sore and painful pelvic tissue internally and externally, using several specialized tools we have developed.

In doing pelvic floor physical therapy, the tightened, irritated pelvic floor can be temporarily released and this sore, painful tissue is put into a kind of "cast," like the cast a broken bone is put in. *This cast is a nervous system cast*—an internal environment in which the sore tissue is not disturbed by the typical bombardment and immune and healing blocking forces of anxiety, protective guarding, reduced blood flow, and the onslaught of insults that ordinary activities of daily life can inflict on the process of pelvic tissue healing. This is accomplished by doing what we call *Extended Paradoxical Relaxation*.

This sore pelvic tissue is continually trying to heal in the pelvic pain patient. These attempts at healing occur in fits and starts—for example, with a good night sleep, hot baths, and daily stress-free time. But these periods of time that support the healing of the tired and chronically irritated tissue of the pelvic floor are routinely short-lived. In general, the pelvic pain patient, in the course of daily life, can't provide sufficient ongoing nervous system quiet, and protection from the irritating bumps and grinds of normal daily life, to permit the irritated and sore pelvic tissue to heal up. As an example, as soon as a good night's sleep begins the healing process for the sore tissue, the next morning the pelvic pain patient is back to the normal grind of daily life and his or her typical levels of anxiety. All of which keep the painful tissue from becoming normal and pain free, as it once was.

It is in the service of providing the painful pelvic floor tissue with a "cast," an undisturbed environment to heal up, that we teach our patients *Extended Paradoxical Relaxation* and ask them to do it from two to four hours a day, in conjunction with regular internal and external physical therapy self-treatment until symptoms resolve.

There is a large literature on the effect of anxiety upon health, wound healing, and the general ability of the immune system to do its work to maintain and restore health to the organism. Below I describe three levels of the inner terrain of nervous system arousal one regularly passes through when doing *Extended Paradoxical Relaxation,* in moving from normal waking consciousness to the zone that supports the healing of sore pelvic tissue.

THE TERRAIN ONE TRAVERSES IN SUCCESSFULLY PRACTICING *EXTENDED PARADOXICAL RELAXATION*

It is useful to talk about three levels of the inner territory one traverses in practicing EPR.

Level 1: Default, Everyday Level of Nervous Arousal

The inner territory I called level 1 is the normal level of tension/guarding/nervous system arousal we live in. It is the default state we inhabit. We walk around, we go to the store, get into a car, sit at the desk, and our inner nervous system engine is going at a speed we tend to regard as normal. When you have pelvic floor pain, you operate in this level 1 state of discernible tension. And when you begin doing a concerted and serious practice of calming yourself down using the method of EPR, you practice letting go of effort, letting go of guarding, letting go of the default level of tension you are used to in level 1. In following the instructions of EPR to let go of effort, you will notice a slight easing of your default guarding, and in doing so you momentarily drop out of level 1 and relax down into what I call here level 2.

Level 2: The State of Maximum Voluntary Relaxation

If you were to say "relax" to yourself and follow this instruction, you would feel a sensation of slight easing, releasing, letting go, and dropping down in your body. This sensation of slight easing, relaxation, and effortlessness is a sensation no different from hot or cold except it is a quieter, more subtle, and easily overlooked sensation. If someone did not direct you to pay attention and cultivate awareness of entering this state in which these subtle sensations exist, you would normally ignore or hardly notice these sensations. The anatomical locations of these sensations of letting go vary and can change over time. Nevertheless *these sensations are the sensations of the release of effort, the un-contraction of muscles.* In level 2, you drop below the level 1 level of default nervous arousal/ tension/guarding into a slightly less tense, but often not particularly satisfying or remarkable, state of slightly increased relaxation that is level 2. This is a state that represents the maximum level of letting go of guiding that you are capable of in the moment.

This happens to be a state that is experienced temporarily when one relaxes to permit urination. During urination, you must relax in order to permit urination to occur. This relaxation recruits the brief, level 2 relaxation of the rest of the body. During this brief relaxation during urination, there may be a momentary, but not profound or lasting, reduction of pelvic pain.

During EPR, it takes earnestness and intention to repeatedly relax in level 2, down from level 1, in order to more or less abide in level 2. At first, the slightest thought can distract the neophyte out of level 2. At the beginning of the EPR session, practitioners drop down for a moment into level 2 and pop right back up into their default level 1 with every distracting thought. This occurs over and over again. Moving into level 2 from level 1, over and over again, is what eventually allows the practitioner to rest in level 2. At first, this often takes one to three hours, especially at the beginning of EPR practice, to come back to the sensation of relaxation and letting go of guarding.

Level 3: Profound Relaxation

And then there is the level under level 2, which I call level 3. My teacher Edmund Jacobson, who was the developer of what's called the *Progressive Relaxation,* implied the existence of level 3 in cultivating the relaxation of what he called *residual tension. Residual tension* is the tension that doesn't easily relax, the level of tension that exists below the level 2.

The level below level 2 is the level of deep nervous system quieting, of deep profound stillness. I consider this state "the healing chamber," the psychophysical state in which the sore and irritated tissue of the pelvis is able to heal.

Level 3 is not something that you can demand to enter, order up, or easily control. Entrance to this state is not obvious and requires a sensibility and practice during relaxation of surrender, nonresistance, nondemand, giving up of attachment to an outcome, patience, and perseverance. Level 3 inner quiet comes to those who paradoxically practice accepting the incomplete and often unsatisfying relaxation level of level 2 until they are then ushered into this often extraordinary experience of level 3. It is the state that occurs when we don't try to manhandle our tension into relaxation or try to beat our pain out of existence. *Level 3 is the deepest level of the experience of no effort.* It is the psychophysical context associated with healing, physical and psychological regeneration and restoration. In yoga it is sometimes called Samadhi. Below is a summary description of these levels.

PSYCHO-PHYSICAL MAP OF THE INNER TERRITORY OF *EXTENDED PARADOXICAL RELAXATION*

EPR Level 1

- Level 1 can be called the normal default level of tension/guarding/nervous system arousal.

- This is the normal level you experience when you are interacting with others, working at your job, driving in the car, talking on the phone, going to the bank.
- It is a state of alertness, the state of being "on," of socially appropriate responsiveness to others and the environment.
- It is a default state you enter when waking up from sleep. It feels like normal, everyday reality. It is generally the state you function in. While the level of relaxation is dynamic in this state, in general level 1 is rarely a relaxed state. When you have pelvic pain, this is the state that the pain often gets worse in as the day goes on.
- When you have pelvic floor pain, you usually operate this state of discernible tension.
- Level 1 is the psychophysical state that you exist in when you are involved in normal discursive thinking.

EPR Level 2

- This is the state you enter into when you ask yourself to relax and then relax as much as you are able to.
- Brief experiences of this level are normally unremarkable, and if someone were not to point out the experience of dropping down into this level, you probably would not take much note of it.
- When you say "relax" to yourself and follow your own instructions, this is the sensation of slight easing, releasing, letting go, and dropping down.
- The physical locations of these sensations in your body can vary and change over time.
- This state is below the level 1 in terms of being in a reduced level of nervous arousal into a slightly less tense, but often not a particularly satisfying state of increased relaxation.
- This is the state of the body one temporarily drops into during urination.
- There is typically little to no change in pelvic pain when first dropping down into level 2, even though it is quieter than level 1.

EPR Level 3

This is a state of profound relaxation that is not able to be accessed by insisting that it occur or the normal method of attempting to calm down. In other words, there is no quick, easy, or simple entrance to this state.

- Entrance to this state is not obvious and requires a sensibility and practice during relaxation of surrender, non-resistance, non-demand, giving up of attachment to an outcome, patience and perseverance and cultivation of successfully focusing one's attention.
- Level 3 is the deepest level of no effort.
- Level 3 is the psychophysical context associated with healing, physical, and psychological regeneration and restoration.

THE MAP IS NOT THE TERRITORY

The words that communicate what to do in order to relax can be called the "map" of the "territory" of voluntary relaxation of the pelvic floor. They are not the "territory." The territory of relaxation, which could be called its skillful practice, can be found only in the depths of many hours of practice.

The words and concepts that describe the practice of what is necessary for the possibility to relax a painfully tensed pelvis and quiet an agitated nervous system happens when one learns to do the following during relaxation practice:

- Understanding the difference between resting in sensation and being involved in thinking.
- Practicing disidentifying with the fearful thoughts and feelings that come into your awareness in favor of being a witness to them and returning attention to the place upon focus.

- Focusing *continuously* on whatever part of your body has been chosen to focus on.
- Accepting tension, which means being willing and able to feel tension/constriction/bracing/guarding in your body, rest with it, and do nothing about it.
- Ceasing to regard as dangerous or bad the discomfort or pain in the area you are focusing on or in the periphery of your awareness.
- Distinguishing tiny amounts of tension contained in the sensation you are focusing on and accept them.
- Be willing to have and accept your experience in the moment instead of trying to have some other experience. In other words, in the moment, practice giving up what you prefer in favor of what you have.
- Earnestly be committed to returning your attention to the chosen site you are focusing on without disappointment, frustration, or remorse for having lost focus.
- Giving up trying to relax; just follow the relaxation instructions and take what you get.
- Giving up trying to achieve anything during relaxation sessions.
- Giving up measuring your progress in the moment of doing relaxation.
- Giving up trying to figure out what is going on in the moment of doing relaxation.

Learning Extended Paradoxical Relaxation
*means repeatedly lying down and practicing the
relaxation instructions outlined in this chapter.*

THE PRACTICE AND GOAL OF EPR IS INTUITIVE AND EASY TO UNDERSTAND ONCE PRACTICE BEGINS

Many of the instructions for this method can at first feel complex and overwhelming to understand and practice. This sense of complexity is found only in trying to decipher the *map* of relaxation training. In the *territory* of relaxation practice, when you are focused inside yourself, these instructions are ultimately simple and clear. However, the catch is that most people feel some fundamental resistance to keeping the mind focused. One must come back to this resistance over and over again, permitting the resistance to paying attention.

RESOLVING PELVIC PAIN MEANS YOU LEARN HOW TO LIVE WITH RELAXED "INSIDES"

The kind of pelvic pain we treat and describe in this book is the result of someone's innards being in an ongoing kind of knot. *Pelvic pain means your guts, your insides, are protectively tight and constricted.* This tightening usually happens simultaneously with the tightening of other parts of the body. It often affects one's breathing, digestion, bowel function, and other aspects of body functioning that are seemingly unrelated.

When you have muscle-based pelvic pain, you live in a body whose core tends to be chronically knotted up.

This chronic knotting up inside, under certain circumstances, can simply let go and one can feel normal again. It is not uncommon for someone with chronic pelvic pain to be on holiday, fall in love, or be released from some major ongoing stress and, in the matter of a few hours, feel almost normal and without pain. Many patients have reported this. Usually, however, the normal circumstances in one's life resume and the old pain and attendant inner contraction reassert themselves.

If you remember peak moments in your life, moments of deep satisfaction and happiness, you may recall that your chest, belly, and pelvis felt good. With the deep relaxation of your body come feelings of hope and love and peace and seeing the goodness in others and in life. A chronically knotted-up pelvis, and sometimes attendant knotting up of the innards of the abdomen, do not allow one to feel peaceful.

Resolving pelvic pain means that we have changed this inner knotting up. It means that our stomach can relax, that we can feel the joy of a complete bowel movement, the relaxation that comes with urination, the deep rest and joy that come after orgasm. It means that our insides are capable of letting go and being relaxed.

> *Resolving pelvic pain means relearning*
> *to live with insides that are relaxed.*

Generally speaking, the state of our pelvic muscles reflects the level of our anxiety and emotional disturbance. Chronic fear and anxiety knot up our insides and tighten our stomach and pelvic muscles. People with pelvic pain who have chronically knotted-up insides tend to get used to inner constriction. This is often because they have experienced it for so long. This inner knotting up feels uncomfortable but normal. Different compensations enter into one's life, trying to calm down one's insides. Overwork, psychoactive and pain medications, substance abuse, overeating, and distractions of various kinds are the common compensatory behaviors in many people with pelvic pain.

Resolving pelvic pain means living life with substantial periods of time when you are not anxious. Usually this means living life with patience, understanding, and compassion for ourselves and others and making the quality of our own life and relationships more important than money, career, or ego. Having a relaxed pelvis means somehow skillfully managing life in the crazy modern world with some degree of wisdom and peace.

CHAPTER 5

THE *WISE-ANDERSON PROTOCOL*, PART 3: UNDERSTANDING HOW YOUR ATTITUDE AFFECTS YOUR CONDITION AND WHAT YOU CAN DO ABOUT YOUR ATTITUDE

Pelvic pain usually does not occur in someone who feels balanced, relaxed, and happy. It tends to be the expression of what is out of balance, fearful, and out of sorts. Your pelvic pain and dysfunction, viewed this way, can be considered an intimate adviser about your life. Pelvic pain is not your enemy. In fact, it is helpful to consider that pelvic pain is part of the main curriculum of your life. Accepting that you have pelvic pain; working to resolve it with kindness and patience makes recovery easier.

Part of the curriculum of pelvic pain has to do with learning to listen to your own body and hear what it is saying: that it needs to be well. Whatever the lessons that are there for you, we believe their resolution can help you heal.

In addition, this chapter will address questions that patients ask about issues including sex, work, relationships, exercise, pain medication, psychotherapy, and alternative treatments, as well as what loved ones can do.

YOU REALLY DO HAVE A CHOICE ABOUT HOW YOU VIEW YOUR CONDITION

A young man with pelvic pain called us from the New York area. He was greatly distressed about his pain and other symptoms. More than anything, he wanted his sexual interest to return, an interest that had waned since the onset of his condition. His anxiety revolved around numerous theories he had read about on the Internet that would condemn him to a life in which he would never get better.

"Do you think this is an autoimmune disease?" he asked, as he quoted some information he had read on the Internet. This young man, like many of our patients, attempted to discover a solution for his problem by reading the literature and the conflicting views and information on the Web.

The theories he read implicating autoimmunity, occult organisms, nerve entrapment, and neurological pathology tended to offer little supporting evidence or effective treatment. They were largely speculative.

His reading made him more anxious and uncertain than before. The more he read that scared him, the more his pain increased. He didn't know what to believe, yet he interpreted his condition from the most hopeless of perspectives, a fear-producing view that offered him nothing while making his condition worse.

Once starting our protocol, a number of our patients decided to stop reading about ideas regarding pelvic pain. "All these theories and speculations about my condition scare me," said one patient. "I have decided not to read any more for now and instead focus on the constructive action I am taking by choosing to begin this treatment." In this way, they were choosing to take charge of how they looked at their condition.

THE PAIN IS NOT THE WORST SUFFERING

The pain is not the deepest source of suffering when someone struggles with chronic pelvic pain syndrome. If we knew for sure that we were going to get better, most pelvic pain and discomfort, while not being something we would choose, would be okay.

*Catastrophic thinking, doubt, and fear
are usually the worst of the sufferings
in dealing with pelvic pain.*

We would most likely put up with it if we did not also experience the kind of angst that attends most people who suffer from pelvic pain. It is the meaning you give to the symptoms that causes the real suffering.

Indeed, the catastrophic meaning one gives to the symptoms and the impact of this meaning on the pain and tension are what is so difficult in dealing with pelvic pain. Consider the following young man, who called us in a state of great anxiety about his condition. He was handsome, accomplished, wealthy, and admired by his peers. Women fell in love with him regularly. His friends loved him. He was successful in his profession. He had it all.

For three years, he had experienced pain at the tip of his penis along with some postejaculatory discomfort and problems with urinary frequency and urgency. The doctors he saw told him that they could find nothing wrong and there was nothing to worry about. He believed them. He characterized these symptoms to himself as an insignificant annoyance and went on with his life with little concern.

He then happened to go on the Internet and started reading the scary stories of those who suffer from pelvic pain, which offered no light at the end of the tunnel. His pain became much worse quickly, and he spiraled into a dark and deeply upset state. His sleep became disturbed. He withdrew socially. He began to worry about others abandoning him because of his condition. His pain escalated from being a minor annoyance to becoming sometimes unbearable. His life became a hell.

This went on for quite some time. Then he found our book, and as quickly as he spiraled into his dark night of the soul he came out of it. He became clear about what was wrong with both him and his symptoms, and his attitude improved dramatically. He came to one of our clinics and his condition further improved. He began having days of no symptoms. Instead of taking a negative spiral downward, in what we describe as the tension-anxiety-pain cycle, he began a positive spiral out of his hole. His view of his condition and its meaning changed. He stopped his catastrophic thinking and saw the possibility of becoming free of symptoms. The ups and downs of his physical pain and dysfunction were greatly influenced by his view of what his symptoms meant.

How you think about your pelvic
pain can strongly affect it.

In his classic book *From Death Camp to Existentialism,* psychiatrist Viktor Frankl observed that while he was in a Nazi concentration camp during World War II he discovered that the one thing the Nazis could not take from him was his choice about how to view things. Frankl was clear in his belief that the way he chose to see things helped him survive. Below we will discuss a strategy to deal with the potpourri of theories and remedies offered to deal with chronic pelvic pain.

The *nocebo* effect—the effect of believing something harmless can hurt you—is relevant here. Theories on the Internet that paint your symptoms as hopeless, theories that are just words and ideas someone proposes—if believed, can be seen as a nocebo and can make your symptoms worse and hijack any quality of life. Many people with pelvic pain walk around miserable for years believing theories that paint a catastrophic picture about their symptoms because they believed things they read on the Internet or ignorant ideas of their doctor.

A PESSIMISTIC VIEW OF YOUR CONDITION CAN LITERALLY CAUSE MORE PAIN

There is scientific evidence demonstrating that your perspective directly affects your pain. Dr. Richard Gevirtz, one of the investigators who discovered that stress increases the level of electrical activity (and pain) in trigger points, described it to me this way: "Where people have a clear-cut model of what is wrong with them and understand that there is something they can do to help themselves, they decatastrophize what is going on within them. This changed view may physically lower their pain by reducing the effects of sympathetic nervous system arousal inside their trigger points. *The source of their pain is not independent of their thoughts and feelings.*"

Is a glass full to the center half full or half empty? In our clinic, we fill a glass of water halfway full (or empty) and ask our participants if the glass is half full or half empty. Most say half full. When asked how they feel about viewing the glass as half full or half empty, unsurprisingly, all say it feels better to see the glass as half full. But as they actually look at the glass of water, it is clear that is equally true to say it is half full or half empty. When we ask our participants what they are looking at when they say it is half full, they come to see that they are looking at the water in the glass being full to the middle. When asked what you would be looking at in seeing the glass as half empty, they come to see that they actually look at the portion of the glass that has no water in it.

In other words, what makes the glass half full or half empty is what you choose to be foreground, what your mind is focusing on. That you can shift your focus from the portion of the glass that has no water to the portion of the glass that has water in it is a real-time demonstration of how what you focus on affects your mood, and your actual experience of pain. Our body listens carefully to our thoughts.

THE SCHOOL OF *COGNITIVE THERAPY*

A school of psychology called *Cognitive Therapy* focuses on helping anxious and depressed individuals identify their habitual negative thinking that triggers or aggravates their depressed or anxious states. From the viewpoint of *Cognitive Therapy,* when there is a choice, you are going to feel better when you see the glass is half full instead of half empty.

CATASTROPHIC THINKING ONLY MAKES YOU MORE MISERABLE AND IS USUALLY NOT TRUE

Catastrophic thinking is a name given to a pessimistic and negative way of interpreting events in which you always imagine the worst. The following example of catastrophic thinking illustrates our point. Imagine you feel a little more rectal discomfort than usual when sitting. From this awareness you think that perhaps the doctor has missed a tumor that might be cancerous. You then imagine having surgery in which they have to remove the tumor. Eventually you die despite the removal of the cancer. You imagine that during your dying no one wants to take care of you and you die alone.

Catastrophic thinking is almost always
a defense against disappointment.

This kind of thinking is not uncommon in many patients that we see. When you tend toward catastrophic thinking, such thinking often feels unremarkable. The catastrophic thinker has rarely considered that there is a real and credible alternative to this way of seeing things. When you think catastrophically, you usually are only dimly aware of the contents of your thoughts, and you only become fully aware of them and their effects after further examination.

Trading possible disappointment for
catastrophic thinking is a poor bargain.

In catastrophic thinking, fear always arises. The thought that something serious is wrong with you sets off an alarm in your body that releases emergency substances like adrenaline and cortisol, readying your body for fight or flight. All of a sudden, your thinking creates a physical event inside of you.

When you began "catastrophizing" about the rectal pain, as we described above, you unwittingly told yourself a story. You jumped from the present moment to four or five steps in the future when you would be diagnosed with cancer. When you have pelvic pain of the kind we describe, these steps that you simply assume will lead you to a diagnosis of cancer are extremely unlikely.

Catastrophic thinking is rarely true and creates needless suffering. The fear of cancer or some other problem that has remained undiagnosed is common with individuals we see who have pelvic pain. This common process of catastrophizing pelvic pain and dysfunction can spin someone into an anxiety state in which the sore tissue–tension-anxiety-pain cycle makes the pain worse and adds misery to the already existing pain and dysfunction. We believe that many visits to the emergency room for pelvic pain occur when catastrophic thinking strongly triggers the tension-anxiety-pain cycle, which then spins out of control.

> *Most people's catastrophic*
> *thinking rarely comes true.*

Ironically, during the writing of this section of our book, we received a call from someone on the East Coast who was in the kind of anxiety state we have been describing. He described himself as "going crazy" as he read the accounts of sufferers of pelvic pain on the Internet who had not been helped and were wretched and desperate. He said his "pain was through the roof." The day after we had an opportunity to discuss our protocol and understanding about the treatment for chronic pelvic pain syndromes, he not only reported that he was feeling relieved emotionally but also expressed his puzzlement because his pain had diminished substantially since our conversation with him. It wasn't our book per se that helped his pain. It was the reassurance he felt in reading it. It is not uncommon for patients we have seen to report a reduction in pain simply from the reassurance they feel that perhaps something can be done to help their condition.

The core treatment we use is aimed at rehabilitating the pelvic muscles, the habit of tensing them, and ultimately the healing of the chronically sore and irritated tissue. However, it is very important to deal with the negative and anxiety-producing thinking that is so typical in patients who have chronic pelvic pain syndromes. People with pelvic pain that we treat tend toward catastrophic thinking, even prior to the onset of symptoms. Changing this tendency is a major life event. Below we discuss issues relating to dealing with the kind of negative thinking that aggravates this condition.

MANAGING THINKING THAT PRODUCES PAIN AND ANXIETY

Understanding that you can't always believe what you think marks the beginning of the ability to manage catastrophic thinking.

What generally can be called *Cognitive Therapy* labels and identifies negative thinking and helps a patient evaluate the credibility of this thinking so that he or she is not a victim of it. For example, using principles of *Cognitive Therapy* a person will think, "I can never do anything right" in response to frustration over making an error. When the person who wishes to gain control of catastrophic thinking becomes aware of the triggering of this kind of thinking, he or she may reflect, "Let me look at the statement 'I can never do anything right' and evaluate whether there is truth in it." Below we share some exercises and processes that we use with patients.

Negative Thought Inventory

The negative thought inventory below is an assessment process that you can use to become aware of the effect of your thoughts on your condition. Choose a three-hour period of time when you tend to feel the worst and pay attention to your thoughts. Use a small tape recorder to record any negative thoughts that occur to you on a minute-by-minute basis. After the thought, choose a number from 0 to 10 as to your level of pain. Some examples of the relevant thoughts include:

- What is wrong with me?
- The pain is worse (maybe it will never get better).
- Am I ever going to get better?
- How can I go on?
- It just does not stop.
- What is going to happen to me?
- Here it is again.
- I can't understand why it is worse.
- Why me?
- Why am I different from so-and-so?
- Will I ever be normal?
- I am never going to get better.
- How can I live my life this way?
- No one will love me like this.
- Maybe I have cancer.
- Maybe I have a sexually transmitted disease and they have not found it yet.
- Maybe I have bacteria or fungus they will never find.
- If I only had not had sex with so-and-so.
- What if I won't be able to function?
- What if I get fired?
- Maybe I won't be able to support myself.

Do your best to record your negative thoughts and their effect on your mood and your symptoms. This may not be the most enjoyable exercise, but it can be instructive in helping you see the frequency of certain thoughts and their effects.

INQUIRING INTO NEGATIVE AND CATASTROPHIC THOUGHTS WITH UNDERSTANDING

Our body responds to the conditions in which we find ourselves. Our body tends to respond to our thoughts as if they were real whether they are or not. A person sees a rope, which triggers the thought that the rope is a snake. This person will likely respond with alarm and anxiety as the body instinctually prepares for the danger of a snake. When he sees that it's actually a rope and releases himself from the idea that it is a snake, his state of alarm stops and his body relaxes.

Cognitive Therapy is not new. It is a general term that refers to the understanding that thinking, in large part, creates the reality we live in. The basic principles of *Cognitive Therapy* are found in an ancient document, the Dharmapada, which states that we create the world we see with our thoughts. If we think we are victims, we ruin our lives. When we do not see ourselves as victims, our lives transform.

Cognitive Therapy is a component of Albert Ellis's Rational-Emotive Therapy, Aaron Beck, former president of the American Psychological Association, and others. *A Course in Miracles* is an existential textbook and a powerful form of *Cognitive Therapy*. For instance, one of the beginning lessons in *A Course in Miracles* teaches that meaning is not inherent in anything. Instead, we give meaning to everything we see. The year-long course offers daily lessons to help students of the course take back control over what they think.

The easiest form of *Cognitive Therapy,* in our opinion, is offered in the work of Byron Katie, who provides an approach to disarming catastrophic thinking by means of a process that one can do oneself. This is the approach we recommend. Her method, which we have adapted to dealing with the negative thoughts around pelvic pain, offers a way of loosening the grip of habitual negative and catastrophic thinking.

Step 1: Finding the Core Thought

The key to disarming the catastrophic thinking related to pelvic pain and dysfunction involves first identifying the core thought that your fear and anxiety rest on.

In Cognitive Therapy, *the core thought is the basic, fundamental thought that is causing us distress.*

Most physicians rarely have the time or inclination to delve into the kinds of thinking that are common to people with pelvic pain. Typically, the person with chronic pelvic pain syndromes at different times lives in a world of negative thoughts that is rarely shared with anyone. Each negative thought is taken in some way to be real by the body as it contracts against the scary world created by the thought. These scary thoughts are like gasoline on the fire of the pelvic pain, inflaming the pain and the cycle of tension, anxiety, and pain and chronic tissue irritation.

The negative thought inventory is a way to identify the core thoughts fueling much suffering in pelvic pain syndromes. The *Cognitive Therapy* process works best with core thoughts that are simple declaratory statements. It is useful to write down these thoughts in the form of sentences. For the question "Will I ever be normal?" the reformulation is "I will never be normal." For the question "Will I ever be able to enjoy sex again?" the reformulation is "I will never be able to enjoy sex again."

It is also useful to take catastrophic thoughts that appear tentative and make them definitive. The thought "Maybe I'm going to be in pain for the rest of my life" then becomes "I'm going to be in pain for the rest of my life."

It takes courage to face a thought that is scary or distressing with an attitude of curiosity and openness.

Both making the negative thoughts into statements and stating them as if they are a certainty are framing them as the body hears them. This reformulation makes the sting of these thoughts easier to identify and deal with when their validity is questioned by this process.

Step 2: Facing the Core Thought with Openness and Curiosity

Like the pain, the negative thoughts are not your enemy. They come from a frightened person's struggle to protect him- or herself. The thought of consciously facing one's negative thinking can appear daunting and depressing. This approach, however, in clearly formulating the core negative thoughts and then examining their validity, usually lightens their impact. In learning to face and evaluate the validity of the negative thinking, one can often soften or neutralize it. It's best to face negative thinking with curiosity and an interest in seeing whether the thoughts are true.

Using Your Heart to Evaluate the Validity of Core Thoughts

It is sometimes useful to experiment with bringing attention to the feeling in your chest and heart area. Feel the breath and the sensation in your chest as the air comes in and out. With your eyes closed and your attention on your heart and chest area, say your name and feel the feeling in the chest. For example, you might say, "My name is John" or "My name is Lindsey" and then you feel the sensation in your chest of truthfully saying your name.

Now keep your attention in your chest area and finish the sentence, "My name is _____," but with a false name. If your name is John, see how it feels in your chest to say that your name is Walter or Dennis. You will probably feel a little tightening or strangeness in your chest. Experiment with feeling your chest as you say your true occupation (e.g., "I am an engineer") and then notice the feeling in your chest when you don't tell the truth (e.g., "I am a baker" or "I am a kindergarten teacher").

The point of Cognitive Therapy *in dealing with
catastrophic thinking is to ultimately release
thoughts that needlessly cause us suffering.*

The point of this exercise is to feel your body's reaction to what is true and what is not true. The body can help you address the validity of your negative thoughts. Refer to the sensation in your body as you address the questions below.

Examining the Validity of the Core Thought

After you have identified the core thought (it is useful to write the thoughts and the answers to the questions down on paper), ask the following questions to yourself about the thought. Feel the area in and around your chest and respond to the questions from this area. In other words, your answers should agree with the feeling in your chest area.

Question your core thought as follows:
1. What is the evidence I have for this core thought?
2. Using this evidence, can I say for sure that this thought is true?
3. What happens physically inside me when I believe that this thought is true?
4. What happens to my self-esteem when I believe that this thought is true?
5. What happens to my experience of my life force, my generosity, and my love when I believe this thought?
6. What has been the effect of this thought or this kind of thought on my life in the past?
7. What would happen to my life if I simply were incapable of thinking this thought or this kind of thought?
8. What is the opposite kind of thought to this one?

We ask our patients to notice the effect of this questioning on their mood and the impact that this thought has upon them. Catastrophic and negative thinking has usually been practiced for a long time. This questioning process can be done often during the day, as these kind of thoughts arise very often. It is possible for this process to help reduce the level of suffering that attends pelvic pain and dysfunction.

> *Catastrophic thinking tends to trigger specific*
> *patterns of tension. When you physically relax*
> *this tension, you can reduce the catastrophic*
> *thinking and its impact on the body.*

Information specifically about this *Cognitive Therapy* work can be found at www.thework.org and in the books of Byron Katie.

GETTING OFF THE INTERNET

We are often asked about other theories regarding the nature of chronic pelvic pain, a subject we touched upon earlier. Many individuals who ask questions about other theories are already anxious and are looking for some kind of reassurance or guidance as to the nature of their condition and the best course of treatment. When they go on the Internet, they read about various theories contending that chronic pelvic pain may be an autoimmune disorder, a condition caused by a trapped nerve, a condition in which occult bacteria are yet to be discovered, or a deteriorating neurological pelvic condition. These theories often tend to promote fear and helplessness in the sufferer.

When you have pelvic pain, it is deeply disturbing to read theories that promote fear, helplessness, and confusion or to hear stories of people who are not doing well with their pain or dysfunction. Some of our patients have asked us whether they should ignore the ideas that they read on the Web or simply avoid the Internet websites devoted to pelvic pain.

In our view, if a theory or an idea about your condition carries some course of action or treatment to help you without unacceptable risks, then it may merit your careful consideration. You may wish to investigate the efficacy of such a course of treatment along with the risks and costs.

> *In general, patients we have seen who*
> *have had the most difficult experience with*
> *their pelvic pain are those who abdicated*
> *their own intuition and judgment in their*
> *decisions about what to do about it.*

If the theory, on the other hand, carries with it (a) *no course of treatment or action* to be done to help or protect you, or if its treatment carries dangers you are not willing to risk, or (b) it offers some *non-definitive* evidence, and (c) it *only helps to create fear, doubt, and disempowerment* in your life, we suggest you tell yourself, "This is someone's theory. There is no definitive proof for it. It offers nothing to help me or protect me, or it carries unacceptable risks. It creates fear and doubt in me. It is okay for me to disregard it as somebody's unproven idea that I will consider if there emerges substantial evidence and/or something to do about it. Therefore I can ignore it as simply someone's unproven idea."

This kind of self-talk is the practice of *Cognitive Therapy*. Using *Cognitive Therapy* about ideas that tend to promote catastrophic thinking is particularly important because anxiety tends to increase symptoms.

> *The best way to stop catastrophic thinking*
> *related to pelvic pain is to be able to*
> *regularly reduce or stop symptoms.*

The core instigator of catastrophic thinking when you have pelvic pain is the underlying thought that there is nothing you or anyone else can do about stopping it. This indeed is the single stilt holding up the catastrophic-thinking house. Over the years we have discovered that when someone is able to reduce their pain, their emotional distress simultaneously reduces. How obvious! In our 2011 study of our Internal Trigger Point Wand, the relationship between the reduction of symptoms and the reduction of emotional distress is very clear. When someone does our protocol, a majority of them can reduce their symptoms. It is for this reason that we say that the best therapy for the emotional distress and catastrophic thinking related to pelvic pain is doing internal and external physical therapy we specify along with *Extended Paradoxical Relaxation*. All of the psychotherapy in the world has little effect on someone with pelvic pain if they cannot reduce their pain and symptoms.

There are psychological interventions that can help in negotiating the ups and downs of symptoms when doing our program, like making a regular list of times in which symptoms are significantly better or absent and then signing each event to document its reality. Indeed it is important to know that symptoms can flare up on the way to a full recovery from them and not "freak out" and go into a full-on catastrophic mode when this happens, but the best solution for catastrophic thinking is to have the experience, over and over again, of symptoms reducing as the result of one's own actions.

FAITH

Faith is usually discussed in church about matters that are spiritual. It is rarely discussed in a doctor's office as part of a medical condition. When you have faith, you have confidence that somehow everything is okay. When you have faith, even though you don't know how things will turn out, you feel assured that you don't have to know. You trust that things will simply turn out all right.

Being willing to have a glimmer of faith
that you will find your way can have
a real impact on your symptoms.

Faith is a frame that you hold up and through which you look at your life. It is an attitude that you bring to situations whose outcomes are not immediately clear. Faith is a willingness to believe that even though you don't see the light at the end of the tunnel, there is light there. The great poet Rainer Maria Rilke wrote to a young poet who was upset about his lack of facility and success in poetry. Rilke told the young poet to *have patience with what was not resolved within him and to embrace the very questions and unresolved issues themselves without trying to figure out answers.* By living in the questions, being fully present in the midst of difficulties (without succumbing to catastrophic thinking), Rilke wrote him, he might *live his way into the answers.*

SUFFERING AS GRACE

Ram Dass was one of the spiritual teachers of young people in the 1960s and has remained a luminary to many since that time. Over the last few decades, Ram Dass proposed the idea that suffering can be seen as grace or a gift. "Suffering as grace" means you acknowledge that even though you wouldn't choose to have the suffering you are dealing with, it turns out to be something that may have in it the possibility of transforming your life.

Usually the awareness that suffering can be seen as grace is perceived after the suffering has resolved itself. Nevertheless, many people who actively have an interest in their inner life inquire as to how their suffering can help them grow and benefit their life.

Ram Dass also introduced a related idea that we have touched upon: that whatever difficulties you may be facing in a particular moment are not distractions from the "curriculum" of your life but the main part of the curriculum itself. Most people believe that their condition has taken their attention away from what they really want to be doing. When you look at your difficulties as your main curriculum, you bring an entirely different attitude to them. This has the power to transform your difficulties, because you stop resisting or hating them.

The deep suffering of pelvic pain is what
prompts our patients to do the demanding
home program we ask them to do.

What does this mean for you if you are suffering from pelvic pain? We are not suggesting in any way that you have deliberately brought this pain into your life, that you want it there, or that you shouldn't resolve it as soon as possible. We are suggesting that if you do have pelvic pain and dysfunction you acknowledge that you have it and consider: What is it asking from me? What lesson does my current predicament contain for me? Am I listening?

TAKING A LONG VIEW: MANAGING YOUR EXPECTATIONS

Unrealistic expectations will make you anxious and increase your pain and suffering. In our view, pelvic pain and dysfunction do not come about out of the blue, even though in some cases they may seem to. It is said that the fruit falls suddenly even though the ripening takes time. In our view someone can have a chronically tight pelvis for years without symptoms and then, with age or certain stresses, the symptoms are triggered. Just as the pelvic pain symptoms don't spontaneously appear, neither do they disappear overnight. In our experience, even with our most successful patients, symptoms take a significant amount of time to resolve.

We suggest that patients who begin our protocol give themselves a good year in which to practice it before expecting symptoms to become reliably better. For those who are helped by our protocol, symptoms usually continue to improve as people practice our method over time (although flare-ups are common with stressful events). Of course, not everyone benefits from our treatment, but for those who do, it usually takes a considerable period of time for symptoms to reliably quiet down.

*When the symptoms begin to improve for
those patients who do well in our program,
these patients typically have "windows" of
symptom relief of an hour, an afternoon, a day,
or a month. Our aim is to help our patients
extend the duration of these windows.*

*Taking a year does not mean that patients will not experience a benefit quite
soon after beginning treatment.* Giving yourself a year means understanding
that typically a person's condition fluctuates, especially at the beginning
of treatment.

We suggest that patients resist celebrating when they are feeling
better or despairing when they are feeling worse. Typically during the
course of treatment they can have twenty or thirty flare-ups, each followed by an improvement of symptoms. Symptom intensity can go up
and down often because it is as if we are renovating a building while still
living in it.

We have touched on the conflict between resting the pelvic muscles
and needing to use them to function in life. In an ideal world, we would
send the pelvic muscles to a tropical island for a long rest. Unfortunately
this is not possible. We cannot avoid the stresses and strains that interfere with our healing and trigger symptoms. We tell our patients to give
their pelvic floor lots of room to go through its gyrations as they do
physical therapy and the two forms of *Extended Paradoxical Relaxation.*

TURNING AWAY FROM REGRET
AND BLAME

We sometimes hear our patients express regret and remorse about sup-
posedly bringing the condition on themselves. These patients often
make themselves miserable with the thought that somehow their current
condition of suffering is one they deserve because they were "so stupid"
or "thoughtless" in bringing the condition on in the first place. Sometimes they say things like "I shouldn't have weight lifted. I shouldn't

have ridden a bicycle. I shouldn't have put myself in such a position of stress. I shouldn't have experimented sexually," among a host of other regrets that patients have expressed.

> *It is neither helpful nor true in any real*
> *sense for pelvic pain patients to think*
> *that they "did it to themselves."*

These particular thoughts are not helpful. They usually serve only to trigger your emotional reactivity, diminish your self-esteem, or produce self-loathing. They keep you stuck in the past, binding up your precious energy in negativity and in feelings of helplessness, because the past is over and what was done is done.

All of us want to be happy. All of us want to be well. None of us would ever do anything to ourselves if we knew at the time it was going to produce a chronic condition of pain. These thoughts are helpful to tell yourself if you are caught up in a cycle of self-regret or self-recrimination.

It may be helpful to tell yourself, "If I knew back then that what I was doing would bring on what I'm dealing with now, I would never have done it, but I couldn't know then what I know now. I can only do my best given the information I have in the moment." Our usual practice with people who have such remorseful, regretful, and self-recriminating thoughts is to help them understand that they were doing the best they could do at the time. An attitude of self-forgiveness is the only attitude that makes any sense and is helpful for the condition. If you can't seem to get your mind behind this kind of thinking, some limited *Cognitive Therapy* can be helpful.

BEING A WITNESS TO YOURSELF

When you have pelvic pain, it usually becomes a major focus in your life. Earlier, we described how we teach our patients in the relaxation training how to be a witness to the experience of tension and discomfort as a way of reducing it and letting it go. Daniel Goleman in his book *Emotional Intelligence* describes being able to be a witness of yourself as an advanced ability to dealing with your own emotions and those of others.

The *Extended Paradoxical Relaxation* taught in our protocol asks that you feel and allow the experience in your body without interfering with it in any way. *As we have discussed, being a witness to your pain and discomfort is usually necessary to relax it.*

> *When you are a witness to yourself, you are able to step outside yourself and look at troublesome thinking and difficult things about yourself without judgment or reactivity.*

DESPERATE PATIENTS USUALLY REGRET DESPERATE DECISIONS

The patients we have seen who have agreed to and later suffered from and regretted heroic measures like pelvic surgeries were for the most part seized by their emotions. In agreeing to these kinds of interventions, they were often in a state of near panic and desperation. "Just do something—anything—to make my symptoms stop" is the message they brought to the doctor. Unfortunately, they often found a doctor willing to participate in their desperate need to do something by experimenting with interventions and surgeries that often left them worse off.

When you are willing to be a witness to your pain and anxiety, you are expressing your faith that somehow it is all right that in the moment fear and pain exist in you. In our experience, in that moment when you allow them to simply be there, they tend to relax. That doesn't mean they all immediately go away. Witnessing tension, anxiety, and pain, however, almost always reduces suffering. As we have examined in the section on *Extended Paradoxical Relaxation,* relaxation occurs with an attitude that it is okay for this pain/discomfort/tension to be here as it is in this moment.

*At the moment you observe you are in a
mental cage, you have stepped out of it.*

Jean Klein, a physician and meditation teacher, noted that at the moment you observe that you are inside a cage you have stepped out of it. Being the witness to yourself allows you to face fear instead of simply reacting to it by fighting or fleeing. When Walter Cannon observed that the reflex response to danger is fight, flight, or freeze, he was commenting on the reflex reaction of the human mammal. When we are willing to witness our unhelpful fight, flight, or freeze reaction, we go beyond our automatic animal programming into a higher domain. Here there is a greater possibility of resolving our concern.

HOW TO GAUGE YOUR PROGRESS ONCE YOU ARE DOING SELF-TREATMENT

Witnessing and understanding flare-ups help reduce their impact. When our treatment works, within a relatively short time there is usually some decrease in the intensity, frequency, or duration of the symptoms interspersed with regular flare-ups.

*With the fluctuating symptoms of pelvic
pain, it helps to remember that you have the
capacity to feel what you feel in your best
moments. In other words, what you feel in your
best moments is what is possible for you.*

Typically a patient will notice an easing in the discomfort of the pelvic floor during or after the relaxation or physical therapy self-treatment, but the discomfort or pain almost always returns sooner rather than later. The "windows" of being pain-free tend to increase, but the course of healing often is three steps forward and two steps backward.

Often patients will feel better for short periods and then return back to the old sense of discomfort and dysfunction. As self-treatment continues, and as the person learns to relax more deeply, the periods of being pain-free and dysfunction-free may increase. Notice if there is a decrease in the *overall* intensity, frequency, or duration of the symptoms. This is a much kinder and at the same time more realistic way of evaluating how your personal healing is going. We tell our patients that they have the capacity to feel as good as the best they feel, and our therapy is aimed at lengthening those good moments and even going beyond them.

PSYCHOTHERAPY CAN SOMETIMES MAKE DEALING WITH YOUR CONDITION A LITTLE EASIER

It is our experience that psychotherapy alone does not significantly reduce or eliminate the symptoms of chronic pelvic pain syndromes. That said, there is a use for psychotherapy in an adjunctive and supportive role in dealing with chronic pelvic pain syndromes.

The anxiety about the future that plagues people who have pelvic pain tends to fester when it is suppressed and is not given a safe place in which to be expressed. When it is painful to sit, to urinate, or to have sex, many thoughts are stimulated about what this all means and what is going to happen in the future. Unexpressed, such thoughts tend to cycle round and round in the kinds of catastrophic thinking we described earlier.

Psychotherapy can be helpful when the psychotherapist has a familiarity with and an understanding of your condition and supports you in what you are doing about it.

It is often hard for most of us to find friends who can hear our fears and anxieties with any degree of understanding and without reactivity. Many people feel baffled, helpless, and afraid to hear about the strange doings and feelings of people who are suffering with pelvic pain. This is one of the important reasons why people with this condition feel isolated and alone. They feel that they have no one to talk to. They are afraid that if they share their real thoughts and feelings with anyone, no matter how close and caring, the person won't know what to do with such sharing. In large part they are right.

Psychotherapy can serve the purpose of having a place to express difficult thoughts and feelings. One of the benefits of psychotherapy is that you are paying someone to be present to hear what is going on, someone who has no history with you.

This kind of psychotherapy can lighten your load a little. When you are choosing a psychotherapist, it is a good idea to find someone who is experienced in treating patients with pelvic pain and who comes recommended. We suggest that patients educate the psychotherapist about their condition by giving them this section of the book to read. When our patients see a psychotherapist after they come to see us, it is sometimes advisable for the psychotherapist to consult with someone on our team to learn more about our protocol and the best way the psychotherapist can support it.

We recommend that patients tell their therapist that they want a place to share their feelings and are not looking for psychotherapy to solve their condition.

Psychotherapists are people. They are as likely as anyone else to deal with their own fears, discomfort, or sense of helplessness upon hearing someone's troublesome situation by trying to "fix" the problem, especially if they have little experience with pelvic pain. This can come in the form of giving advice or making global psychological interpretations about the meaning of the symptoms. Such psychotherapeutic interventions, in our view, are entirely unhelpful and are to be avoided.

A NOTE TO FAMILY AND FRIENDS OF SOMEONE WHO HAS PELVIC PAIN

It is not easy for the loved one of someone who has pelvic pain. The caring spouse, child, parent, or friend of someone who has pelvic pain usually goes up and down emotionally with the person dealing with pelvic pain, and we have been asked on more than one occasion if we have any advice for him or her. Here are some thoughts.

The pelvic pain that we describe in this book is not life threatening. It is not a progressive disease that eats away at someone like cancer. People with pelvic pain do not have a shortened life expectancy because of it. While symptoms can be intense, and in some cases make the normal activities of work and other aspects of life very difficult, symptoms tend to wax and wane.

> *The idea that the pain will never go away is the*
> *real suffering in chronic pelvic pain syndromes.*

If people with pelvic pain knew that they were going to be out of pain in a week, the pain and dysfunction they deal with would usually be more tolerable. They would just wait it out with the expectation of its going away. It is the idea that it will never go away, that they will never be able to be free of pain, that is the real suffering of this condition. In other words, the catastrophic thought is the real suffering. Similarly, if the loved one or friend knew that it was going to be over, the physical pain and dysfunction would be more like your loved one having a cold, and there would be the clear expectation that the cold would certainly be over.

But when the doctors don't help pain and dysfunction that go on and on without the hope that they will stop, and the person in pain is depressed and anxious, the experience of pelvic pain can be a real psychological and spiritual crisis for both the patient and his or her loved ones. When people suffer, their loved ones suffer along with them.

The dilemma of those who are close to someone with pelvic pain is that they know that the person they care about is suffering and in pain, but they feel there is nothing they can do. It is this feeling of helplessness that is so difficult for both the patient and the loved one or friend of the patient. Sometimes loved ones or friends feel they have to do something, yet they find that there is nothing to do. They want to reassure the person, yet they really don't understand the problem and don't know what to say. They don't know if everything will be okay. Those who are close to someone with pelvic pain often feel guilty thinking how their loved one's suffering limits their own life and the way it affects them. The suffering of the pelvic pain patient is usually a lonely suffering, with no one who understands the problem and no one to help. The suffering of the loved ones of the pelvic pain patient is equally lonely. Often they suffer for years alongside the patient with no one to really talk to and with no idea about what to do.

If you are a pelvic pain patient's loved one or friend, it is helpful to let go of the thinking that you are somehow responsible to solve the problem.

What can the loved one of a pelvic pain patient do? While there is no quick and easy answer to this question, we have a few thoughts. Being close to a pelvic pain patient requires a certain kind of psychological and spiritual development and maturity. If, in some way, you are related to someone with pelvic pain, we think it is helpful to remember that ultimately the solution to your loved one's difficulty is not in your hands. You are not responsible. It is helpful to remind yourself that someone dealing with pelvic pain must find his or her own way and that you can simply be loving and understanding without having to figure out or solve the problem. In other words, with kindness and love, it is often helpful to let the person with pelvic pain have the problem. Undoubtedly, if you could fix the problem you would. But you can't. In the end, it is not yours to solve. This is not easy to hear or practice. Under the circumstances, however, it will be most helpful to the person you're close to with pelvic pain if you don't burn out with frustration and depression about feeling helpless.

The friend of a pelvic pain patient once reported that he was in the hospital room of his cousin, who was hooked up to machines that were monitoring his vital signs. He noticed that he tightened up inside when the numbers on the machine were not the numbers he wanted to see for his cousin. He eased up when the numbers were more to his liking. His tightening up, he realized, was a kind of irrational attempt to control the numbers. In his desire for his cousin to be well, he unconsciously, irrationally thought that if he tightened up and resisted the "bad" numbers, they might be more likely to change to the good numbers. He realized after a few hours of doing this that he was emotionally and physically exhausted. He became aware of the impossibility and irrationality of trying to control the readout of the machines he was watching and realized that if he continued this inner game of inwardly resisting the numbers he didn't like he would wear himself out and not be able to be emotionally there for his cousin. And of course, nothing positive would be accomplished. He decided to abandon this game he was playing and instead *inwardly permit the numbers from the machines to be whatever they were*, accepting them and not trying to fight them. He found this was the most helpful thing he could do to help his cousin.

> *If there is nothing you can do about*
> *your loved one's condition, feeling guilty,*
> *frustrated, or depressed about the condition*
> *won't help you or your loved one.*

This story can be instructive to the loved one of someone with pelvic pain. Doing everything that you can do yet also *permitting the situation inwardly, not arguing with reality, in our view is the best way to deal with the difficult situation of pelvic pain.* Practicing acceptance of what is going on in the moment as it is and not projecting that it is necessarily what the future will hold, not feeling guilty for it, not taking responsibility for it, and being willing to do whatever can be done but allowing for the fact that the solution for the problem is out of one's hands are all helpful ideas both to the loved one and to the patient.

In this way, being in a relationship with someone you love who has discomfort or pain, but whose condition you can't change, is really a practice in accepting what is. You have to deal with your own catastrophic thoughts about your loved one's condition. In fact, both you and your loved one don't know what the future holds. But the tendency of many people who are close to those with pelvic pain as well as those with pelvic pain is to go to the catastrophic conclusion that it will never be better.

Catastrophic thinking is a challenge to deal with for both the person with pelvic pain and the loved one of such a person. We deal with the issue of having a loved one in pain in the same way as we deal with other matters in our lives. Practicing the art of noticing catastrophic thinking, evaluating its validity, and extricating yourself from its grip is essential in being close to someone you love who may have pelvic symptoms.

You can practice accepting your loved one's
situation as it is in the moment without
projecting that it will always be that way.

Most individuals who deal with pelvic pain don't appreciate being asked all the time how they're feeling. A continual, worried question of "How are you feeling?" can strain, frustrate, and shame someone who is dealing with the symptoms we describe in this book. If you are a loved one of someone with pelvic pain, it is often better to specifically ask that person whether they want you to ask them how they are feeling. If they say, "If I want to share how I'm feeling at any particular moment with you, I will. Otherwise, it's better not to be asking me how I'm doing," in our view it is best to heed this kind of request. Let pelvic pain patients be responsible to take care of their situation and be responsible to share how they are feeling, if this is what they wish. This kind of open dialogue is often helpful.

Other practical things can be done. If your loved one comes to a clinic of the *Wise-Anderson Protocol* and you and your loved one are willing, you can learn trigger point release methods that may be of benefit to your partner. In general, what quiets down someone's nervous system helps them. You can offer to do foot massage or neck and shoulder massage or hold them if that is helpful to them. This is often very much appreciated by the person with pelvic pain. You can listen to the fears and suffering of your loved one and practice permitting your loved one to have these thoughts and feelings without joining your loved one with your own fearful and catastrophic thinking.

If you are close to a pelvic pain patient, take care of yourself. In the airplane, we are instructed to put our own oxygen mask on first before even putting the mask on our children. Similarly, make sure you are getting enough "air." Make sure that you are taking care of yourself. If your life is upset, you tend to become an additional burden for your loved one with pelvic pain.

We have helped many people with pelvic pain help themselves. We are very optimistic that those with pelvic pain can learn how to substantially reduce or resolve their symptoms. Sometimes pelvic pain goes away spontaneously. This condition can get better. It can go away, and even when there is a flare-up, when patients know how to treat themselves it can be a nonevent. That is certainly one of the goals of the *Wise-Anderson Protocol*. In summary, if you are close to someone who has pelvic pain, it is best to take care of yourself, be loving and available for your loved one, and see the current situation as an opportunity to be present with what is going on in the moment without jumping to some kind of conclusion that you can't know is true.

EMDR

Besides cognitive and supportive psychotherapy, some forms of psychotherapy can be used for more specific purposes. One such approach is eye movement desensitization and reprocessing (EMDR) for sexual and physical trauma.

A small but not insignificant number of patients have tightened their pelvic muscles chronically as a reaction to physical or sexual abuse. Often they did so as part of their way of defending themselves against the trauma reoccurring. "If I open myself up and relax, I will be inviting something bad to happen so I have to remain contracted" and "If I open myself up, I will be overwhelmed by the pain inside me" represent the kind of unconscious thinking of some people who have experienced trauma-related pelvic pain.

> *EMDR is a method of choice in dealing with*
> *physical or sexual abuse associated with pelvic pain.*

We generally refer patients who have had sexual or physical abuse that may be contributing to their pelvic pain to a psychotherapist experienced in EMDR. This method aims to resolve frozen feelings and memories from abuse that occurred at a time in the person's life when such feelings and memories were impossible for the person to process.

Dr. Francine Shapiro discovered that earlier traumatic events seem to loosen their hold on traumatized people when, in a therapeutic environment and guided by a trained therapist, they move their eyes (or attention) rhythmically while talking about the event. EMDR makes use of the fact that parts of the body connected with processing of experience tend to freeze up during a traumatic event and remain frozen.

> *EMDR helps unfreeze a person's frozen*
> *consciousness and the mechanisms of*
> *catharsis around a traumatic event in order*
> *to process and resolve the event internally.*

To understand this, recall what you do when you have had a difficult encounter during the day. Typically you will want to talk about it and share it with someone close to you. You do this as a way of "processing" the difficult experience in order to be able to let it go so that you can be free in the moment again. Imagine what would happen if you had a fight with your boss, your spouse, or your friend that was not resolved and you were very upset but you were not able to talk about it with anyone. The experience would feel like something stuck inside you that needed to come out but could not. Being unable to share your thoughts and feelings would most likely feel extremely physically and emotionally uncomfortable.

Those who have been victims of incest, sexual trauma, or physical assault feel a level of distress multiplied by many orders of magnitude in comparison to a simple interpersonal upset. Consciousness tends to freeze during this kind of event as if to control or contain it. The traumatized person perceives the trauma to be too big to handle, and as a result, his or her body and mind freeze up around the trauma to protect the self from being overwhelmed.

The methodology of EMDR allows the event to be processed in the same way you would process an upset with your boss by talking to a friend. The processing that occurs in EMDR around traumas such as sexual and physical abuse or physical trauma such as some kind of painful surgery or procedure, however, tends to be much more dramatic than your discussion with your friend about the upset with your boss. Tears, shuddering, grief, and anger can arise in the EMDR processing. Such reactions were suppressed during the traumatic event. As the event continues to be recalled while the eyes, ears, or senses focus on rhythmic movement, the trauma can be processed and resolved.

CATHARTIC PSYCHOTHERAPY

Any difficult life situation that does not allow a person to express strong emotions or feelings can result in a person chronically tightening the muscles of the pelvic floor. For instance, we have seen patients whose triggering event appears to be the suppression of grief around the death of a loved one or some other life-shaking loss. We speculate that the pelvic floor muscles are tightened because the emotions are not being expressed and the ongoing nervous system arousal chronically flares up pelvic floor–related trigger points.

> *Catharsis-oriented psychotherapies can be of use in helping our troubled patients vent suppressed emotions. In this way, a major obstacle to treatment can be removed.*

Several psychotherapeutic methods are useful in allowing suppressed emotions to be expressed. Reichian therapy, bioenergetics, rebirthing, and Holotropic Breathwork are all methods that have grown up on the periphery of standard "talking" psychotherapy. They are methods that aim specifically at providing an environment and methodology that can assist a person in directly expressing emotions that have been suppressed.

Wilhelm Reich, M.D., the inventor of Reichian therapy, was particularly interested in what he called the muscular "armoring" of the pelvis and the effect of stopping the energy and feeling from moving through it. Reich developed a powerful psychotherapy able to unlock suppressed emotions.

Cathartic therapies like bioenergetics and Reichian therapy help restore someone's ability to express deeply distressing emotions.

Alexander Lowen, M.D., a New York psychiatrist, popularized Reichian therapy in a form called bioenergetics. Lowen wrote several popular books from the 1950s through the 1990s. Bioenergetics is also very effective in dealing with suppressed emotions.

Stanislav Grof, M.D., developed Holotropic Breathwork as a way of reconstituting the therapeutic aspects of the psychedelic experience without the use of drugs. Grof is a researcher who studied psychedelic substances and was deeply moved by the power of these drugs to produce positive therapeutic effects. Holotropic Breathwork is often done in groups, lasts a number of hours per session, and encourages patients to let down and allow their deepest feelings to arise and be expressed. This too is a powerful methodology.

A full presentation of the theoretical underpinnings and methods of Reichian therapy, bioenergetics, and Holotropic Breathwork is beyond the scope of this book. We believe these modalities can be useful in helping to express and sometimes resolve emotional difficulties that some of our patients may have that interfere with their relaxation of the pelvic muscles.

SEXUAL SHAME, GUILT, AND FEAR

The issues of shame, guilt, and fear with regard to sex sometimes may be related to pelvic pain and are appropriate subjects to be dealt with in psychotherapy that is adjunctive to our protocol. Numerous studies have demonstrated a higher incidence of pelvic pain among women who have been sexually traumatized. While studies have not focused so much on men, in our experience issues around sex are often related to the onset of pelvic pain. Let's explore briefly the likely relationships among sexual anxiety, shame, guilt, and pelvic pain.

Those with chronic pelvic muscle tension tend to tighten up during the experience of sex as a way of defending themselves against feeling the vulnerability and intimacy of the sexual experience.

The pursuit of sexual pleasure, the frustration humans often experience in achieving it, the turmoil that often attends it in interpersonal relationships, and the religious injunctions against it are all issues that loom large in human life.

Without lowering nervous arousal that feeds chronic pelvic tension, physical treatment alone can be like pressing on the gas pedal with one foot while pressing on the brake with the other.

Here are some examples. We saw a forty-year-old woman who had been raped by her father when she was fifteen. Her core belief was that the only way for her to be safe was to not allow anything to come into her vagina again. Twenty-five years later she came to see us because she was suffering with vaginal pain. Of course, a central focus of our treatment was teaching her to relax her pelvis. Her traumatic history, however, fought against the goal of our treatment.

Usually core beliefs exist unconsciously in individuals who, like this woman, have experienced sexual trauma and related pelvic pain. These beliefs must be addressed before our protocol can be fully effective. A prominent EMDR therapist reported working with a young woman who had been raped by her father when she was three and who held the belief that if she relaxed her vagina her insides would fall out. Others hold the belief that the only way to protect against the heartbreaking violation of rape or sexual assault is to live with a tight and guarded pelvic floor. Again, this psychological dimension must be addressed if patients are to give themselves permission to relax their pelvic muscles.

We also saw an eighteen-year-old man who was nervous about sex. Remarkably, he had never masturbated or had any sexual activity in his life. He began having intense sexual dreams, which frightened him, and he tightened up his pelvic muscles as a way of trying to control the sensations and emotions that were arising. After several months, he went to his family doctor and reported having problems with urinary frequency and urgency and pain above the pubic bone. This man's core belief was that if he permitted himself to feel his intense sexual feelings he would lose control of himself, and that belief deeply frightened him. Asking this young man to relax his pelvic muscles without helping him resolve his sexual anxiety would not be a viable therapeutic strategy.

These examples represent a small percentage of our patients. Nevertheless, for certain patients these issues are crucial, and resolving them makes it possible for symptoms to abate.

PLEASURE ANXIETY: WHEN FEELING SAFE FEELS SCARY

Psychotherapy can be a useful adjunct when addressing what can be called "pleasure anxiety." Pleasure anxiety refers to an aversion toward pleasure because it triggers an unconscious fear that something bad might happen if one is happy and unprepared for danger. Pleasure anxiety is often seen in individuals who have suffered some life-changing trauma, like the death of a parent.

Pleasure anxiety can reach the level of terror in some individuals, and the relaxation protocol must be modified to help someone through this anxiety. Very occasionally, as people with pleasure anxiety follow the relaxation instructions and the nervous system begins to quiet down, their hearts begin to beat faster, their palms begin to sweat, and, to their distress, they feel more anxious doing relaxation. This reaction is simply a heightened psychological defense against letting down their guard and vigilance.

> *Pleasure anxiety is a fear that being*
> *unguarded and enjoying yourself leaves you*
> *vulnerable and unprepared for bad things.*

While this kind of reaction prompts someone having it to stop doing relaxation, on the contrary perseverance through this reaction is vital—but instead of fighting the defense, one must be gentle with it. Sometimes it is necessary to reduce the duration of the relaxation session to a period of one or two minutes so that the subconscious can discover that it is safe to quiet down, even for this short period. As one can tolerate more time of reduced arousal, one increases the duration of the relaxation session. It is a delicate dance, and the sufferer needs to rely on someone who understands what is going on and can guide the sufferer through it.

Here is an example to explain pleasure anxiety. A patient with pelvic pain experienced the suicide of her mother at a time in her life when our patient was happy and carefree. The news of her mother's death occurred suddenly and shocked her. From the time of her mother's death she remained nervous and wary. In her mind, the experience of being happy and carefree was somehow connected to a terrible event happening.

It was for this reason that she complained she could never relax. With a psychotherapist, while in therapy, she had noticed that as she grew older and explored her life she seemed to be uncomfortable "feeling good." She reported that invariably when she felt a sense of contentment, negative thoughts about things that might happen in the future would come to her mind and her good mood would evaporate. Moreover, she reported that she felt strangely naked when her pelvic pain would subside. Her treatment involved a focus on tolerating pleasure and accepting the absence of anxiety. This was no small enterprise.

> *Our treatment bumps up against*
> *psychological patterns that refuse to let go*
> *of guarding against imagined danger.*

The core of our treatment for pelvic pain is training our patients to profoundly relax their pelvic muscles. You can't relax the pelvic muscles without relaxing everywhere else in the body. *Extended Paradoxical Relaxation* means that you "un-defend yourself." It means that you allow yourself to be at ease, to feel good, and to let go of vigilance.

When patients are at a plateau in which their symptoms stop improving, it is often helpful to facilitate a dialogue between the part of the patient who wants to improve and the part that seems unable to move ahead. What often emerges from these dialogues is the fear of the unknown that is imagined if there is no more pain or dysfunction.

PROSTATITIS AND SEX

But in abacterial prostatitis/nonbacterial prostatitis/CPPS, which represents approximately 95 percent of all cases, sexual functioning and pleasure are often affected. If the symptoms in chronic pelvic pain syndrome are intermittent, generally speaking, sexuality is affected only when other symptoms are present.

When symptoms are experienced either intermittently or chronically, many men have discomfort during or after ejaculation. Typically, a man diagnosed with abacterial prostatitis/nonbacterial prostatitis/CPPS experiences increased aching, discomfort, or pain after intercourse lasting from a few hours to a few days. This experience takes its toll, and while most men continue to experience sexual desire, it is dampened by the sense that there will be pain or discomfort afterward.

> *It is common for some men to complain of a*
> *reduction in sexual interest, problems performing*
> *sexually, or a diminution in the strength of*
> *their erections. We do not believe that there*
> *is a physical basis for these complaints.*

Though the responses of the spinal cord reflexes are dampened by pelvic discomfort, it is our view that the man's attitude and emotions and/or anticipation of pain can also have a powerful effect on the reduction of sexual interest, pleasure, and functioning.

COMPULSIVE SEXUAL ACTIVITY AND PELVIC PAIN

Some individuals deal with their anxiety and depression by engaging in compulsive sexual activity and masturbation. Anxiety and depression briefly disappear during orgasm. This disappearance is almost always short-lived. The great rise in the availability of pornography on the Internet is a possible factor that has rarely been taken into account in the treatment of pelvic pain of certain individuals. At this time we have no idea of the number of men who fit into this category, although anecdotally it appears not to be a large number. Nevertheless, it is a subject that deserves discussion.

> *Pelvic pain can be triggered and exacerbated*
> *by compulsive sexual activity.*

It is a common experience that repeated orgasms in close proximity yield diminishing levels of pleasure. The diminishment of pleasure with frequent orgasm also yields diminishing relief from anxiety and depression. It is not well known that compulsive sexual activity and pornography will tend to make anxiety and depression worse and not alleviate it. Someone indulging in compulsive masturbation in an attempt to relieve anxiety or depression is not unlike someone in Las Vegas who wins a big jackpot at a slot machine and then continues to play the same slot machine in the hopes of getting another jackpot, even as the payouts become smaller and smaller.

One of the things that happen when you use orgasm and compulsive sexual activity to fight depression and anxiety is that the pelvic floor is forced continually to strongly contract and relax during orgasm. This often pushes the prostate, seminal vesicles, and pelvic floor muscles to overwork. When the frequency and level of intense contraction of these muscles are sustained beyond a certain point, the pelvic pain may be triggered. If the syndrome is already present, compulsive sexual activity will often exacerbate it.

> *Forcing an already tight and painful pelvic*
> *floor to frequently contract through compulsive*
> *masturbation will tend to make pelvic pain worse.*

Very frequent orgasm triggers or exacerbates feelings of anxiety or depression and pelvic pain by making the pelvic floor muscles bear the burden of using orgasm as a kind of antidepressant strategy. During orgasm, there is a transient reduction or absence of pelvic pain, depression, and anxiety. When symptoms of psychological malaise are soon felt again and the urge to feel better through orgasm arises, and masturbation is engaged in, orgasm can momentarily make anxiety and depression again calm down. One of our patients said that he could reliably eradicate his feelings of anxiety completely during and in the first few minutes after orgasm.

In the book *Cupid's Poisoned Arrow,* Marnia Robinson discusses the notion that masturbation and orgasm prompt a surge of dopamine. She goes on to describe the theory of how, after the brief dopamine surge, the release of prolactin along with other brain changes can lower the state of the pleasure of the orgasm and can foster a sort of anhedonia, or pleasureless state. Nevertheless, the desire to feel better in someone who compulsively masturbates reasserts itself, and repeated masturbation both yields less pleasure and creates more physical and psychological malaise.

> *Stopping the addiction to pornography and*
> *compulsive masturbation can help reduce*
> *the intensity of pelvic pain symptoms.*

It is recommended in *Cupid's Poisoned Arrow* that someone who has been engaging in compulsive masturbation, sexual activity, and/or use of pornography and who comes to realize the importance of stopping such compulsive, addictive behavior should abstain from ejaculation for a period of two to four weeks or longer. Robinson proposes that this period of time helps rebalance the person's two-week cycle of disturbance after orgasm. From our view, it can help calm down pelvic muscles that are continually caught in the vise of postorgasm hypertonicity. *Cupid's Poisoned Arrow* is an excellent discussion of the effects of compulsive sexual activity and its remedies.

IF YOU GIVE UP COMPULSIVE
SEXUAL ACTIVITY, HOW DO YOU
FIND PLEASURE AND RELEASE?

In the absence of compulsive and addictive sexual activity, joy, satisfaction, reward, and pleasure must be found elsewhere. Perhaps what is most important is that the individual find another way to calm down anxiety and reduce nervous system arousal. Using our protocol, it is possible to reduce anxiety and nervous system arousal with both the deeply relaxing effect of internal and external trigger point release and the quieting of an aroused sympathetic nervous system using *Extended Paradoxical Relaxation*. Social interaction, friendship, creative pursuits, exercise, and other activities that bring meaning and quality into one's life are also needed to replace what is sought from the effect of compulsive sexual activity.

A "middle way" must be found to replace the intense, supernormal kinds of stimulation of orgasm induced by pornography. The relief and pleasure of *Extended Paradoxical Relaxation* can be an important substitute for the relief of compulsive sexual activity.

> *The reward of competence in* Extended
> Paradoxical Relaxation, *beyond helping to reduce*
> *or stop symptoms of pelvic pain, is the routine,*
> *deeply felt pleasure of profound relaxation.*

Extended Paradoxical Relaxation can be what you call on to feel balanced and at peace, a feeling you once sought in vain from intense sexual stimulation. As Robinson describes in *Cupid's Poisoned Arrow,* one often goes through a real withdrawal when reliance on masturbation/pornography-driven orgasm is stopped.

WHY THERE IS INCREASED DISCOMFORT AFTER SEXUAL ACTIVITY

It is very common for men with prostatitis/chronic pelvic pain syndrome and for women with pelvic pain/pelvic floor dysfunction to experience increased discomfort or pain hours or the next day after orgasm. This increase in discomfort during or after sexual activity in men and women with chronic pelvic pain syndromes occurs because orgasm causes strong contractions of the pelvic and, for men, prostate and seminal vesicle muscles lasting about one a second during orgasm.

Dr. Jeannette Potts observed that *orgasm is a pleasure spasm.* There is a significant increase in nervous system arousal during sexual activity. The pleasure spasm of orgasm in the form of an increased series of contractions during orgasm will tighten the pelvic muscles further. This increased tightening temporarily contracts an already contracted area that doesn't relax well, and it tends to throw the patient further above the symptom threshold. After a while, the muscles relax and return to their baseline level, and the normal state of the pelvic floor reasserts itself (returning to some degree of pain or discomfort when a person has chronic pelvic pain syndrome). For this reason we do not recommend increasing sexual activity when a person has a pronounced increase in symptoms after sex.

REDUCING POST-ORGASM-RELATED SYMPTOMS

In general it is better to reduce the frequency of sexual activity when one has muscle-related pelvic pain. And with sexual activity continuing, it is important to quiet down post-orgasm-related symptoms.

Toward this end, it is sometimes helpful to do stretching and trigger point release of the anal sphincter, coccygeus, anterior levator, and other pelvic floor muscles after sex, whether by skin rolling, self-massage, or the insertion of a gloved and lubricated finger inside the pelvic floor. It is also often useful to do relaxation before sex or relaxation and a hot bath after sex. Some patients have escaped the flare-up of sexual activity by taking Valium or Klonopin before or immediately after sex. The point of all of these strategies is to quiet down the tightening of the muscles after sexual activity and to restore their ability to relax after the strong workout of orgasm. These strategies become less important as the pelvis returns to a more overall relaxed state and an unirritated state.

INCREASING NONSEXUAL INTIMACY IN THE MIDST OF THE PAIN AND DYSFUNCTION OF PELVIC PAIN SYNDROMES

Men in our culture tend to be uncomfortable in acknowledging either to themselves or others their needs for closeness, connectedness, and nonsexual intimacy. In our culture men often slap each other on the back, punch each other on the shoulder, or call each other names to express their affection and connection with each other while maintaining the appearance of appropriate manliness.

Often anxious men who are not in a sexual relationship will frequently masturbate as a way of lowering their anxiety. *In a word, sex is often used by men to address needs that are not sexual.*

> *For many men, sexual intercourse is one of the only ways they find that they are able to receive love, affection, closeness, and reassurance.*

When men have some form of chronic pelvic pain syndrome, they must bear many burdens that are not discussed. Men we see in our clinic frequently complain of their reduced interest in sex. What they rarely express, however, is that when they have pelvic pain and dysfunction, often discomfort related to sexual activity casts a pall on one of the only ways they can be intimate or relax.

When sex is particularly difficult or onerous, we recommend to our patients to choose to cuddle with their partner without the aim of being sexual and having orgasm. These intimate yet nonsexual moments can address a man's often increased anxiety and help reduce the tensions that may be present in the marital relationship.

> *If sex hurts, it is okay to be less sexual for a while—not to stop sex but to reduce its frequency until one is more regularly able to reduce the tension in the pelvic floor after orgasm.*

Not uncommonly, some men with prostatitis have an idea that their masculinity depends on their ability to have intercourse and satisfy their partner. When we suggest that perhaps they have sex less frequently, these patients may express discomfort and worry at how their partner will react.

We will sometimes suggest that our patient be clear with his partner that he can give her sexual pleasure but will refrain from having orgasm himself. This pleasure might be in the form of sexual massage, or bringing his wife to orgasm without having intercourse. In this way the strain on his relationship, which is often a big concern to our patients, can be softened while the chance of a flare-up of symptoms is minimized.

NONE OF THESE MEASURES IS IDEAL: THE BEST SOLUTION IS FOR THE CHRONICALLY SORE PELVIS TO HEAL

We do not want to give the impression that simply cuddling or pleasuring one's partner resolves the sexual issues brought about by pelvic pain syndromes. These measures are attempts to ameliorate the situation under circumstances that are, at best, difficult. We understand that the best solution we can offer to the issue of sex and the problems that arise between men or women with chronic pelvic pain syndromes and their partners is for them to be able to help themselves reduce or stop their symptoms.

Relaxing during sexual activity can help
calm down postorgasm discomfort.

We have found that entering into and completing sexual activity while the pelvic muscles are relaxed can help reduce discomfort related to sexual activity. Below we will outline some steps you can take in changing the often unconscious habit of tensing the pelvic muscles before and during orgasm.

BECOMING AWARE OF WHAT GOES ON IN YOUR PELVIC MUSCLES DURING SEXUAL ACTIVITY

Here are some notes on relaxation related to sexual activity.

- Notice if you are anxious in anticipating being sexual.
- Notice if any anxieties occur during sexual activity.
- Notice if there is any sense of urgency in moving toward orgasm or if there is a sense of leisure about it.
- Notice if there is any unnecessary tightening of your pelvic muscles as sexual sensation builds up, as you get close to orgasm, or during orgasm.
- Do your best to notice if you add unnecessary tension to the experience of sexual sensations.
- Notice what happens when you practice the intention of voluntarily reducing your tension during sexual activity.
- Notice if there is any difference in the quality of the orgasm or in your level of discomfort after orgasm when you slow down and relax during sexual activity.

Relaxing the pelvic floor during sexual activity usually means slowing down and relaxing to feel the sexual sensation over and over again if there is a tendency to reflexively tighten against its intensity.

The instructions of *Extended Paradoxical Relaxation* can be used to change the habit of overly squeezing the pelvic muscles during sex. Your practice of *Extended Paradoxical Relaxation* will be most clearly seen in your ability to accept and relax with the incompleteness of the sexual experience midway through it. Men commonly are captured by the impulse to get to the orgasm. This impulse is usually accompanied by pelvic tension and lack of ease. Our recommendation is: instead of tightening your pelvic muscles and rushing toward orgasm in the way that you might normally be accustomed to do, slow down and feel the subtlety of the sensations along the way.

Doing this is not easy at first and requires a certain discipline and willingness to postpone immediate gratification. We will address below the subject of not making sex an emergency.

It is helpful for someone with pelvic pain to not
treat coming to orgasm as an emergency.

When a man has a high level of tension in his pelvic muscles, it is common that he tightens up during sex. Anxiety about performance and "rushing" to the climax are not unusual. When a man squeezes his pelvic muscles at a time when the pelvic muscles naturally contract, there is often a reduction in sexual sensation and more likelihood of increased discomfort afterward.

For this reason we offer the idea of not making sex an emergency. What this means in practical terms is that a man practices the relaxation method of our protocol throughout his sexual experience. This means that he stays in touch with his often unconscious tendency to tighten his muscles during sex and, instead of reflexively tightening, relaxes.

Relaxing during sexual activity means that
you allow the genital experience to come
to you rather than trying to control it.

This practice of relaxing during sex is unknown territory to most men. Doing this requires being receptive more than being active. It means that anxiety is not in the driver's seat during the sexual act. Relaxing during sex tends to be accompanied by an increased level of physical and emotional sensitivity.

Being in a sexual embrace while being profoundly relaxed is not a new idea. This attitude has been around for thousands of years and exists today in the practice of what is called tantric yoga. While tantric yoga has spiritual goals, our purpose in discussing this practice is to help restore the health of the pelvic muscles and reduced strain during sex.

It is important that sex not be an emergency situation. Having sex in a relaxed way in conjunction with the rehabilitation and relaxation of the pelvic muscles helps keep the pelvic muscles from going into the heightened level of tension that we believe is responsible for increased discomfort after intercourse.

> *Learning to deeply relax during sex often takes time, patience, and perseverance. Aside from reducing symptoms, this practice has other rewards of increased presence, intimacy, and pleasure.*

GUILTY OR ANXIOUS SEXUAL PAIN (GASP)

A small but distinct group of men complain of pelvic pain consistent with the typical diagnosis of prostatitis or chronic pelvic pain syndrome that arises after they have experienced a sexual encounter that they later regard with shame, guilt, or regret. In this discussion, we will refer to *guilty or anxious sexual pain (GASP)* from such an encounter.

Typically in this scenario, a man will pay a woman for a sexual massage, engage a prostitute for intercourse, have a casual or long-term affair outside marriage, or engage in some other variety of sexual activity about which he retrospectively feels anxiety or guilt.

Commonly, after the sexual encounter, the man fears that he has contracted an STD because of adverse symptoms. All appropriate tests are conducted and no STD is found. In the urological and psychological literature, there is little to explain the relationship between prostatitis/CPPS symptoms and the sexual behavior involved in the encounter. We suggest here that men who report GASP tend to have a common psychophysical response to their behavior that results in the perplexing symptoms of prostatitis/CPPS.

Chronic prostatitis/chronic pelvic pain syndrome for a small number of male patients is associated with sexual guilt or anxiety about a sexual encounter.

PSYCHOPHYSICAL MECHANISM IN GASP

Contemporary urologic theory has been less than enthusiastic about implicating psychosocial factors in the onset of urologic disease. A mechanistic, body- and organ-centered explanation of the varieties of urologic pathology pervades the urologic literature. Here we are proposing a psychological theory of how psychosocial factors are intimately involved in the causation of symptoms of prostatitis/CPPS.

We are suggesting that a person's attitude and psychological viewpoint can result in a physical reaction in a man with GASP-induced pelvic pain/dysfunction. This man tends to operate with a rigid moral outlook. *Events in life tend to be perceived as black or white, right or wrong, good or bad.* He applies this moral standard both to others and to himself. There tends to be little room in his mind for events, feelings, and behaviors to be objectively viewed as they are, without a moral label. He tends to disown feelings or behavior that he judges to be bad or wrong and regards himself with contempt and rejection.

> *Men whose onset of pelvic pain occurs after*
> *a guiltily or anxiously perceived sexual*
> *encounter tend to be hard-pressed to forgive*
> *feelings or behavior in themselves or others*
> *that they judge to be bad or wrong.*

Typically a man with GASP-induced pelvic pain views the sexual event retrospectively with remorse, guilt, and fear of having violated a moral code, being discovered by his partner, or having contracted some kind of disease. When we questioned such men about the reasons for their behavior, there was little self-understanding about how they had allowed this sexual encounter to occur. When in a relationship, they tended to show no forgiveness of the circumstances and context in which such an event occurred (e.g., they were lonely, sexually frustrated, estranged from their partner, or in need of some kind of relief, reassurance, or self-esteem that was lacking). Instead, when asked about the behavior, the response of these men was "It was wrong and I shouldn't have done it and I feel guilty and afraid because of it." It was also not uncommon for them to say, "I probably deserve what I have."

Men with GASP tend to give themselves little psychological space to have erred. We propose that their pain and dysfunction is the result of a twofold attempt to punish themselves and to control themselves into refraining from such behavior in the future. They do this by tightening the muscles of the pelvic floor to stop the sexual feelings there from overwhelming them and causing them to lose control of their behavior. Elsewhere we have discussed the theory that pelvic pain is the result of chronically pulling the tail between the legs, and is associated with fear, shame, remorse, or guilt. It is not uncommon for a dog to pull his tail between his legs when his owner expresses upset over the dog's behavior.

> *On a psychological level, men with pelvic pain*
> *associated with a sexual encounter would do*
> *well to ultimately forgive themselves and come*
> *to understand that they can control their sexual*
> *impulses without tightening the pelvis.*

In other words, we are suggesting that the primary purpose of the response of these men to their own behavior that they reject in themselves is to chronically tighten their pelvic muscles as a way of stopping their sexual sensations in order to control their behavior. As in other men with muscle-related pelvic pain and dysfunction, this chronic tension and guarding creates an inhospitable environment in the pelvic floor that results in pelvic pain and dysfunction. In summary, guilt about sexual encounters leads to fear about self-control. The resultant unconscious prolonged tightening is aimed at controlling sexual impulses and sexual acting out.

We treated an accountant with GASP. He reported that during tax season, a period of significantly increased stress in his life, and while at odds with his perfectionistic and judgmental wife, he had an affair with the secretary of one of his partners. He expressed great shame over his behavior, as he considered himself a morally upright and religious man. He said that his moral values would never permit his infidelity, but somehow he did it anyway. His affair went on for a little over a year. His wife discovered his infidelity and he went through a period of anguish with her. They sought counseling and he expressed his remorse repeatedly during their counseling sessions, promised never to do this again, and begged his wife's forgiveness.

Things more or less went back to normal in his relationship, but it was at this time that his pelvic pain began. Initially when asked whether he had experienced any intimacy, stress reduction, or beauty in his extramarital relationship, he could not find any value in it. He had difficulty focusing on the question of whether the affair served him in any way. He appeared not to want to appreciate what he got from the affair and instead repeatedly returned to his self-judgment and self-condemnation. Upon reflection, he reluctantly admitted that his extramarital affair had brought him comfort, pleasure, self-esteem, and stress reduction but quickly reiterated that these benefits could not justify his behavior.

Shame and guilt in GASP patients may be accompanied by the biological response to chronically pull the tail between the legs.

He had great difficulty in conceiving that he could forgive himself for his behavior. When he was asked what he imagined would happen if he forgave himself for his infidelity, he answered that if he forgave himself he just might go back and do it again.

Men with GASP whom we have seen tend to have difficulty in differentiating between thought, feelings, and behavior. When we proposed that it was possible to allow the experience of sexual feelings without acting on them, men with GASP tended to be perplexed. How you allow impulses and emotions to be present while not acting on them was a strange concept to most of them. And yet this distinction is critical for men with GASP if they are to give themselves permission to relax their pelvic floor.

Our theory about this patient and others with GASP is that, in their shame and fear about their behavior, they pull their tail between their legs continually and cannot imagine stopping doing this. This chronic tightening of the pelvic muscles is their way of ceasing to feel their sexual impulses. Not feeling their sexual impulses is their way of controlling them, thereby controlling acting on them.

The *Wise-Anderson Protocol* for GASP

We are proposing that there is a psychological requirement for a man who wants to overcome his GASP and related pelvic pain/dysfunction. He would do well to forgive his behavior and come to understand that he can have a relaxed pelvis and feel sexual feelings and that he does not have to chronically tighten up his pelvic floor muscles in order to control his sexual impulses. He would probably help himself by coming to understand that a relaxed and uncontracted pelvic floor will necessarily open up the experience of sexual feelings and that these feelings are natural and one need not judge them as wrong or bad in order to control acting on them.

Typically men with GASP and related pelvic pain/dysfunction disown their experience, as they consider it bad or wrong. *This psychological disownment occurs simultaneously with the tightening of the muscles of the pelvic floor.* When this disownment is added to an idea that their bad or wrong behavior should be punished as a way of controlling it in the future, they unconsciously tighten their pelvic floor even more.

Once this period of chronic pelvic tightening occurs, as in other men with muscle-related pelvic pain, the condition takes on a life of its own. This condition is fed by the cycle of tension, anxiety, pain, pelvic muscle irritation, and protective guarding. Added to that cycle, in these particular men, is protective guarding against sexual feelings that arise in the pelvis. In summary:

- Men with GASP tend to operate in a right-wrong world and judge what they perceive as their own morally wrong behavior with contempt and disownment.
- This disownment is both a psychological event of repudiation and judgment of their behavior and a physical event of imple-

menting this disownment and repudiation by physically chronically tightening up the pelvic floor.

Treatment of GASP

Psychological treatment of GASP requires the modification of both the self-contempt and the thoughts that say, "The only way I can control myself is by tightening up my pelvic muscles as a way of controlling my sexual acting out." The man has to feel that it is okay to have sexual feelings, that it is okay to have a loose pelvis and to experience sexual arousal, and at the same time to understand that he can control sexual impulses without killing the experiencing of the sexual impulses. It goes without saying that the full protocol we offer, including physical therapy and *Extended Paradoxical Relaxation*, must be an integral part of treatment.

PHYSICAL EXERCISE AND CHRONIC PELVIC PAIN

The relationship between exercise and pelvic pain is not often addressed. Little written about this subject, even though many of our patients are anxious for advice about whether to initiate, continue, or stop physical exercise.

> *The kinds of physical exercise that are most likely to aggravate symptoms of pelvic pain and dysfunction when someone is symptomatic include weight lifting and bodybuilding, sit-ups, crunches, and bicycling.*

We think that bicycling aggravates symptoms in some people because it pushes on the tender, painful trigger points in and near the perineum. These often highly trigger-pointed and tender areas are not happy being pressed upon by bicycle seats.

Weight lifting and bodybuilding have been associated with the onset of pelvic pain in a number of patients we have seen. A few patients who undertook a crash course in flattening their stomachs reported that their pelvic pain began after their regimen of five hundred sit-ups per day got into full swing. While all exercise causes a contraction of the pelvic muscles, sit-ups and weight lifting, demanding the abdominal muscles to strongly contract, put a large burden on the pelvic muscles. It is not surprising that this kind of exercise can initiate or aggravate pelvic pain and dysfunction that arise from chronically contracted muscles.

There are doctors who insist that when the pudendal nerve is compressed, one must protect it by avoiding exercise like bicycling or rowing, which tend to aggravate it. While pudendal nerve entrapment remains a controversial and speculative general explanation of chronic pelvic pain, if one is symptomatic, avoiding exercise like bicycling or rowing is a harmless precaution.

Sometimes, therefore, certain physical exercise is contraindicated. Patients who have enjoyed or benefited from these types of exercise ask us whether they should resume these exercises in spite of their increased pain, or whether they will ever be able to go back to them. Our view is that some kinds of physical exercise can aggravate pelvic pain because they put a strong demand on the pelvic muscles to contract—muscles that are already shortened because of chronic tension. These tensed, shortened muscles don't relax very well. When physical exercise tightens them further, they remain in an elevated state of tension for a while. For reasons upon which we can only speculate, some people's symptoms are affected while others' are not.

Some patients diagnosed with prostatitis, interstitial cystitis, and urethral syndrome have reported that certain kinds of exercise worsen their symptoms while other kinds do not. Others report that they feel better after exercise. Still others report that exercise has no effect on their symptoms. Certain practitioners have insisted that no one with pelvic pain should lift weights or ride a bicycle.

We think such pronouncements are unduly restrictive. If a patient has irritation or inflammation/ulceration in the bladder or urethra or experiences flare-ups after bicycle riding or weight lifting, then obviously the patient needs to be selective about his or her mode of exercise. But if no tests indicate problems in the bladder or urethra and if the patient does not notice any untoward effects in doing weight lifting or bicycle riding, in our view there is no reason to give them up.

Our general advice to our patients about
physical exercise is to find a form of cardiovascular
exercise that minimally exacerbates their
symptoms.

If bicycle riding does not exacerbate one's symptoms, or if one's symptoms in the area of sitting have cleared up, we think it entirely reasonable for someone who loves bicycle riding to experiment with bicycle riding to see if it is workable for him or her. If he or she notices symptoms related to this activity, then common sense says to curtail such an activity. If no symptoms occur, we see no reason to banish bicycle riding or other activities that have been routinely discouraged by some who treat pelvic pain.

Unfortunately, more than a few individuals who come to see us feel that exercise might hurt them. We have had patients who have stayed in bed for months because of their idea that exercise would hurt their condition. But in general, physical exercise lowers levels of anxiety and is beneficial for the body in numerous ways.

HATHA YOGA AND STRETCHING

Part of our protocol in the physical therapy component of our treatment involves doing stretches to loosen the muscles in the pelvic floor that have been shortened. These are specific kinds of stretches aimed at assisting with the rehabilitation of the pelvic muscles, and we include these exercises as part of our homework for the patient.

The muscles of the pelvic floor can be stretched to some limited degree. We believe the program of external stretching that we previously described is the best for lengthening and loosening contracted pelvic muscles. It is a kind of yoga.

> *While yoga postures can be helpful for pelvic*
> *pain, postures that require tightening up the*
> *pelvic muscles may be postures to avoid.*

Hatha yoga is an ancient practice of physical stretches that are called "asanas," or postures, aimed at relaxing the body and preparing it for meditation. The popularity of yoga has grown in the West, and in many places yoga studios are as common as coffee shops or nail salons. We support hatha yoga, as we see it helping the muscles to stretch and lengthen as well as helping the body to quiet. If patients have little free time, we encourage them to do the stretches described in this book that are specifically aimed at the lengthening and relaxation of the pelvic muscles.

The only caveat we offer with regard to yoga is that it be done with plenty of time to relax in between poses. Furthermore, we do not recommend yoga that requires prolonged awkward poses that tighten the pelvic floor up.

MASSAGE AND BODYWORK

Whatever calms you and soothes you is good for pelvic pain. Full-body massage, while sometimes costly and time consuming, is a very good activity for someone who has pelvic pain. Swedish massage, shiatsu, Rolfing, Esalen massage, Jin Shin Jyutsu, Reiki, Rosen bodywork, Feldenkrais, Trager, craniosacral therapy, tui na, and reflexology are all types of bodywork that usually have the effect of relaxation and quieting. A number of our patients have unsuccessfully sought out these approaches as a primary treatment. In our view, none of them has any lasting benefit for pelvic pain. Nevertheless, we consider them useful in quieting down anxiety and nervous system arousal.

MEDICATIONS FOR PELVIC PAIN AND DYSFUNCTION

We know of no curative medications for the kinds of pelvic pain and dysfunction described in this book. While there are generally no effective pain medications, some medications can "take the edge off" the pain on a temporary basis for some patients.

For some patients with intolerable symptoms, pain medication must be used. All medications for pelvic pain, however, have varying degrees of effectiveness, typically come with significant side effects, and in our view rarely offer a satisfactory resolution of symptoms.

In general there are no really effective medications to deal with chronic pelvic pain. It has been our experience that alpha blockers like Flomax, Hytrin, Cardura, and Uroxatral can offer modest relief to some patients with pelvic pain but can cause considerable side effects for some patients, including nasal stuffiness, elevated heart rate, dry mouth, and fatigue. Elavil, originally used as an antidepressant, at certain dosages is sometimes prescribed in nonantidepressant doses for pelvic pain.

Perhaps of all the medications that have a limited efficacy for discomfort in the pelvis, the benzodiazepines like Valium or Klonopin can help give the sufferer a "break" from the discomfort. Sometimes patients will take 2 to 2.5 milligrams of Valium every four hours for a day or two or 5 or 10 milligrams of Valium every third or fourth day to help sleep and to reduce the constant discomfort or pain. Patients should exercise caution about addiction and sedation with these medications and should consult with their physicians about their use.

While narcotic medications can reduce pelvic pain, complications to these drugs include addiction, lowered pain threshold, a need to increase medication over time, constipation, and general mental dullness. Some of our patients have a harder time getting off the narcotics than they do in releasing their pain. In general, when possible, we would discourage the use of narcotic medication. But we can work with people who are on narcotic medications, even though these medications tend to complicate treatment to some degree.

> *While narcotic medications are sometimes the only way in which someone can tolerate pelvic pain, our physicians do not prescribe these kinds of drugs.*

PELVIC FLOOR BIOFEEDBACK

The following discussion was written by David Wise, Ph.D., and edited for this edition, as a response to a question on the Internet about the usefulness of pelvic floor biofeedback:

> I am responding to a request for a comment about the usefulness of intrapelvic biofeedback measurements in determining if pelvic pain is a tension disorder and appropriate for the *Wise-Anderson Protocol*. My short answer is that electromyographic measurement of the anal sphincter and/or muscles near the opening of the vagina with a biofeedback sensor, used alone, is generally an unreliable measure of what is going on inside the pelvic floor. Unremarkable readings of the anal sphincter and/or vaginal opening should not be used to rule out tension-related pelvic pain or to dismiss the appropriateness of the *Wise-Anderson Protocol*.
>
> Here is the longer answer. Let me say first that I have been a biofeedback supporter and practitioner for over twenty-five years. I had the best of training over many years from one of the luminaries of the field and have worked with many patients over the years with multimodal biofeedback for anxiety, functional cardiac disorders, and urinary incontinence, among other problems. I continue to do neural feedback training with Steve Wall, one of the geniuses in the field of biofeedback and the designer of the remarkable biointegrator system. In addition, I did biofeedback assessment and

training in intrapelvic biofeedback at Stanford for a number of years with many patients.

We have found that pelvic floor biofeedback
is usually not helpful for muscle-based pelvic
pain and in certain cases can exacerbate it.

Biofeedback that measures skin temperature, galvanic skin response, muscle tension, brain wave activity, and respiratory sinus arrhythmia for problems other than pelvic pain is remarkable and enormously helpful. Our view about biofeedback not being useful relates specifically to pelvic floor biofeedback for chronic pelvic pain syndromes that we discuss in our book in which a sensor is inserted rectally and/or vaginally and readings are measured on an electromyograph in microvolts. It does not refer to intrapelvic biofeedback for urinary incontinence, which I happen to think is the best and safest treatment that exists for incontinence or for other uses of biofeedback that have been of great benefit to many.

In my own case, when I was symptomatic, I did an hour or two of pelvic floor biofeedback on a daily basis for a year. After many months of diligent practice, my resting anal sphincter tone was a remarkable zero after about fifteen minutes of relaxation. And I was very dismayed, like the person whose comment you sent to me, to find that I was still in pain at the moment that the anal sensor registered zero. I was also disappointed as a clinician experienced in the successful use of biofeedback for other problems to find that the biofeedback measurement seemed to indicate (erroneously) that tension was not a central problem in my pelvic pain.

I didn't understand then what I understand now, which is that the electrical activity in the anal sphincter and/or vaginal opening is, for the most part, the only area that the biofeedback sensor measures, and often says very little about what is going on with the other twenty-some muscles within the pelvic floor and external muscles related to pelvic pain. Furthermore, the biofeedback sensor measures dynamic muscle tension but not chronically shortened tissue without elevated tone. It is possible to have a relaxed anal sphincter and/or vaginal opening and have pain referring pelvic floor trigger points deep inside that can make one very miserable. In this case, elevated tone and active trigger points inside the pelvic floor are not reflected in the anal sphincter and/ or vaginal opening measurements.

There can be a normal biofeedback reading at
the opening of the vagina or anus while painful
trigger points exist in the pelvic floor muscles.

Shortened, contracted tissue inside the pelvic floor, symptom-re-creating trigger points inside and outside the pelvic floor when palpated, the habitual tendency to tighten the pelvic floor under stress or to reflexively guard against pelvic discomfort, and a tension-anxiety-pain cycle are the culprits in most people with pelvic pain that we successfully treat. This can sometimes but not necessarily include a chronically tight anal sphincter and/or vaginal opening. All of these factors are diagnostically significant. For example, in my experience at Stanford, people with levator ani syndrome almost always have an entirely normal resting anal sphincter tone while the painful trigger points on the levator and other internal muscles are palpated. Resolving those trigger points and relaxing the inside of the pelvic floor can resolve this pain without much change in the measurement of the tone of the anal sphincter before or after treatment.

On our website, www.pelvicpainhelp.com, we have video clips of an important study, replicated many times, demonstrating that at rest the electrical activity inside a trigger point in the trapezius, monitored by a needle electromyographic electrode, is quite high while the electrical activity of the tissue less than an inch away from the elevated electrical activity is essentially electrically silent. If you used a regular biofeedback sensor to measure the general tone of the trapezius, you might well find nothing remarkable, yet to rely on this information would be entirely misleading and would incline you to miss the treatment that could substantially reduce or abate the pain and dysfunction coming from the active trigger point.

The best person to evaluate muscle-based pelvic pain after any pathology is ruled out is someone experienced in trigger point release and myofascial release inside and outside the pelvic floor.

The bottom line here is that in my experience electrical measurement of the anal sphincter and/or the opening of the vagina, used alone, is often a poor measure of what is going on inside the pelvic floor. While I believe biofeedback is remarkably successful for many other disorders and is one of the treatments of choice for urinary incontinence and vulvar pain, I am unimpressed with the usefulness of biofeedback in treating most pelvic pain.

The best gauge of the usefulness of our protocol that treats pelvic pain of neuromuscular origin is a thorough examination of the pelvic floor for trigger points that re-create symptoms and palpation for tightened and restricted muscles inside the pelvic floor. This must be done by someone with a significant amount of experience in working with pelvic pain and with the kind of myofascial trigger point release and relaxation methods that we use. An inexperienced person will miss all this, and I have seen many times that even practitioners who specialize in treating pelvic pain miss trigger points referring the symptoms to and inside the pelvis.

We sometimes find pelvic floor electromyography useful when there is a high pelvic floor resting tone because it provides an objective marker that we can compare readings to after the patient has used our protocol. The idea that pelvic floor biofeedback measurements are a reliable test of whether pelvic pain is a tension disorder represents a misunderstanding of the problem and should not be relied on, especially when the readings are normal. Pelvic floor electromyographic measurement monitoring the anal sphincter and/ or the vaginal opening is one of those medical tests where a positive finding may mean something and point toward the proper therapy and a negative result doesn't necessarily prove anything.

MONITORED KEGEL EXERCISES

When we wrote the fifth edition of this book, many patients who spoke to us reported that they had done pelvic floor biofeedback as a treatment for pelvic pain. Pelvic floor biofeedback usually involves doing Kegel exercises (tightening the pelvic muscles as if stopping urination and then relaxing the pelvic muscles). This alternation typically is done for five to twelve seconds of tightening and then five to twelve seconds of relaxation.

We generally believe that Kegel exercises are not useful with pelvic pain and, in fact, can exacerbate symptoms. Kegel exercises were developed to help women restore their continence after childbirth. They are exercises to strengthen and tighten muscles, not to relax them. Kegel exercises usually add tension to an already tense area in someone who has pelvic pain. While Kegel exercises can be very useful for women who have vulvar pain or incontinence, we generally think they are contraindicated for pelvic pain.

USING THE *WISE-ANDERSON PROTOCOL* FOR OTHER MANIFESTATIONS OF PELVIC TENSION

The consequences of chronically holding tension in the body are not limited to pelvic floor pain and dysfunction. A modified *Wise-Anderson Protocol* may be useful in other conditions that arise from chronically holding tension in the body, such as constipation, anal fissures, hemorrhoids, irritable bowel syndrome, and post–bowel movement pain.

One of the larger conclusions of our book extends an idea that we have quoted earlier, namely that the development of a solution to any difficult problem is often not found within the confines of the field designated to study it. The basic tools of conventional medicine in general and the specialty of urology in particular confine themselves to pharmaceuticals and surgery. Certainly pharmaceuticals and surgery have revolutionized modern civilization and have extended the life span and health of humankind. But in the case of pelvic pain, though the diagnostic tools of urology that rule out structural pathology are essential, the therapeutic tools of drugs or surgery have not helped and sometimes have actually complicated or exacerbated the problem.

The protocol we describe in this book may be
helpful for a variety of conditions related to
the lower abdomen and the pelvic floor.

CONSTIPATION, ANAL FISSURES, AND HEMORRHOIDS

Constipation is sometimes associated
with symptoms of pelvic pain and
sometimes exacerbates them.

The colon and rectum are structures that operate together to evacuate stool. Normal bowel elimination involves a complex mechanism that includes the reflex relaxation of the internal anal sphincter when the rectum is full. This sensory muscle, which is autonomically controlled, can differentiate between gas and stool and signal the pelvic floor muscles to relax if it is appropriate to eliminate (along with appropriate peristalsis in the colon). However, if it is not socially appropriate or convenient, an individual can voluntarily tighten up the pelvic floor and help quiet down the sense of urgency that is felt.

Heightened anxiety can lead to increased tension in the pelvic floor. This interferes with the ability of the muscles to release at the appropriate time, at the same time disturbing normal peristalsis in the bowel. There are also individuals who have learned to do the opposite of what needs to be done in order to eliminate. Instead of relaxing their pelvic floor muscles, especially the puborectalis muscle, they contract it while attempting to eliminate, causing a frustrating condition called paradoxical puborectalis contraction. Fortunately this condition is relatively easily diagnosed and is reversible with neuromuscular reeducation. It is important to stop the habit of this paradoxical contraction, as prolonged bearing down can result in prolapsing pelvic or abdominal organs.

An anal fissure is like a paper cut in the mucosal lining of the anal sphincter. Many researchers call it an "ischemic ulcer." Ischemia is a condition of significantly reduced blood flow to an area. The current understanding about anal fissures is that because there is elevated tension, the blood flow in the anal sphincter is reduced, thereby impairing the tissue, which then becomes fragile and vulnerable to injury from a hard bowel movement or from the pressure of bearing down during defecation.

> *Anal fissures usually occur in the presence of a highly contracted anal sphincter. One of the benefits of the* Wise-Anderson Protocol *is that it can help many soften and relax a chronically tightened anal sphincter without drugs or surgery.*

It is generally agreed that the cause of the anal fissure in large part involves a chronically tightened internal anal sphincter. Surgery, the procedure of stretching or dilating the anal sphincter under anesthesia, and the application of topical agents to the internal anal sphincter are aimed at relaxing the anal sphincter. The rationale for surgery on anal fissures is based on the peculiar idea that cutting the sphincter is the best way to reduce the tone, tension, and spasm in the anal sphincter. While surgery can be successful, there is some risk of short-term and sometimes long-term fecal incontinence.

At some time or another, many people find a little blood in their stool, usually after a particularly hard bowel movement. They can become confused and upset at such an event. At other times, alarmed individuals go to the doctor complaining of rectal pain after a bowel movement with no apparent blood in the stool. Often the doctor gives the diagnosis of anal fissure or hemorrhoids to these complaints. Hemorrhoids constitute another condition that is painful and sometimes the source of blood in the stool. A hemorrhoid is a kind of varicose vein that tends to balloon out when one is straining on the toilet.

One French study showed that one-third of women had hemorrhoids or anal fissures after childbirth. This is probably because of the great pressure exerted by bearing down during childbirth in addition to the prevalence of constipation during pregnancy. Millions of people in North America suffer from hemorrhoids. Anal fissures and hemorrhoids are common in both men and women. These conditions are often related to constipation and diarrhea. Constipation has been related to chronic tension in the pelvic muscles in adults and recently to refractory constipation in children in a study done at the Mayo Clinic.

While most anal fissures and hemorrhoids resolve themselves after they flare up, some colorectal surgeons lean toward an aggressive procedure or surgery to treat hemorrhoids and anal fissures. We have seen patients who are anxious about their rectal discomfort talked into treatment of the fissure or hemorrhoid involving surgery.

Conventional treatment of constipation, anal fissures, and hemorrhoids tends to ignore the relationship between body and mind.

Like the literature on the conventional treatment of pelvic pain, the literature on treating constipation, anal fissures, and hemorrhoids almost entirely ignores their relationship to a person's mind-set, level of relaxation during bowel movements, and management of stress. Instead, there is a narrow focus on immediately reducing symptoms of these conditions. Procedures, surgery, laxatives, and medications are the usual options.

Most of the patients we have seen who have had surgery for anal fissures or hemorrhoids have reported that the physicians they saw offered few options related to quieting down the anxiety and habitual straining and tightening related to these conditions. Instead of seeing an anal fissure, for example, as an expression of anxiety and chronic pelvic tension, conventional treatment sees its symptoms, including chronic anal tension, as something that needs to be mechanically or pharmaceutically stopped. Little regard is shown for the big picture of a person's life and how one's symptoms are a response to this big picture. It is our view that the symptom is the way our bodies are trying to communicate. If we refuse to understand the message because we don't understand the body's language, we needlessly suffer and don't deal with the root problem prompting the symptom.

In the large majority of cases, chronic tension in the pelvic floor, including the anal sphincter, usually combined with diet, anxiety, and time urgency around bowel habits, strongly contributes to constipation, anal fissures, and hemorrhoids. The chronic pelvic tension, diet, and bowel habits associated with most constipation, anal fissures, and hemorrhoids do not come out of the blue. In a word, a person's mind, body, and lifestyle are involved in the creation and perpetuation of these conditions.

We propose that a modified *Wise-Anderson Protocol* might be of significant benefit for the treatment of constipation, anal fissures, and hemorrhoids. The overriding principle is that all of these conditions tend to occur as the result of expressing anxiety by tightening the pelvic floor, and in the case of constipation, inhibiting normal peristaltic movement in the colon.

This can be accomplished by teaching patients the trigger point release and *Extended Paradoxical Relaxation* protocols we use for pelvic pain syndromes.

A devoted effort of self-treatment in the *Wise-Anderson Protocol* that we teach in our six-day clinics, we believe, might be of help for someone suffering from constipation, anal fissures, and hemorrhoids. Of course, the modification of the *Wise-Anderson Protocol* would have to include diet and bathroom habit reeducation, teaching the patient not to strain unduly and not to resist the feeling of urgency to go to the bathroom.

IRRITABLE BOWEL SYNDROME (IBS)

IBS is common in the general population and is reputed to be the most common disorder in visits to gastroenterologists. The symptoms of IBS typically include abdominal pain, abdominal bloating or fullness, diarrhea or constipation, sometimes heartburn, early feelings of fullness, and incomplete bowel emptying. Typically it is treated with certain medications, avoidance of colon-irritating food and drink, increased intake of water and fiber, and exercise. It is a distressing disorder and often comes and goes with periods of stress.

Treatment of IBS with a Modified
Wise-Anderson Protocol

In our six-day pelvic pain clinics, a number of patients who also suffer from irritable bowel syndrome have reported improvement in their IBS symptoms. These patients have reported that this improvement occurred after they did a specific kind of abdominal self-treatment to be discussed below, in combination with *Extended Paradoxical Relaxation*.

What follows discusses the treatment and a proposed mechanism to explain the possible efficacy of this modified *Wise-Anderson Protocol* for IBS. We do not advise someone to use this method for these conditions without physician instruction and supervision, since if one does not understand abdominal anatomy and the appropriate pressure to be used, blood vessels and structures in the abdomen can be damaged.

Irritable bowel syndrome used to
be called spastic colon.

IBS is common in both male and female patients whom we have treated for pelvic pain. The purpose of the *Wise-Anderson Protocol* is to teach patients targeted self-treatment methods. One of the methods we now show patients is that the use of the Trigger Point Genie allows them to easily do abdominal trigger point release. Some of our patients with IBS had dramatic improvement of their symptoms of abdominal or esophageal discomfort when they exerted trigger point release pressure to areas of tenderness or pain throughout their abdomen. This was done in conjunction with the regular practice of *Extended Paradoxical Relaxation.*

Proposed Mechanism of the Modified *Wise-Anderson Protocol* on IBS

In their classic book *The Colon,* Stewart Wolf and Harold G. Wolff observed that in patients with abdominal fistulas (open holes in the abdomen) that permitted direct visual examination of the colon in different emotional states, the colons of the subjects studied tended to become slowed down and contracted (hypodynamic), stopping their rhythmic movement, during periods of fear, dejection, futility or defeat, dissatisfaction, boredom, tension, and mild depression. The subjects' colons became hyperactive (hyperdynamic) in moments of anger, resentment, guilt, humiliation, anxiety, and conflict. When the emotional states of these individuals became quiet and calm, the colonic behavior normalized and the rhythmic peristaltic movement and color resumed. Wolf and Wolff stated:

> In the patients described, it was common to find a disturbance of colonic function characterized either by a hyperdynamic response with diarrhea, or a hypodynamic response with constipation. Hyperfunction was characterized by hyperemia, a contraction of longitudinal muscles together with shortening of the colon and increase in rhythmic contractile activity of circular muscles in the caecum, ascending, and transverse loops while the descending and sigmoid colon showed no rhythmic circular contractions but assumed a rigid tubular shape due to longitudinal muscle activity, with pallor of the mucosa. In colonic hypofunction with constipation, rectal, anal and perianal muscles were usually contracted so as to further impede emptying.

. . . The hypodynamic reaction was encountered when individuals reacted . . . with feelings of fear, dejection, futility, or defeat, dissatisfaction, boredom, tension and mild depression . . . sustained or recurrent colonic hypofunction in patients was found to be associated with constipation . . . may be looked upon as a part of a general reaction of "grimly holding fast" under circumstances that threatened the individual.

The hyperdynamic reaction of the colon, on the other hand . . . [was related to] symbolic assaults which included anger, resentment, guilt, humiliation, anxiety, and conflict. Catastrophic or shocking situations or those arousing feelings of being overwhelmed also evoked hyperfunction of the large bowel. . . . [This can be called] the ejection-riddance pattern of colonic hyperfunction.

Early in the twentieth century Walter Cannon, originator of the terms *fight, flight, freeze* and *homeostasis,* noted a similar reaction in the colon of a cat that rhythmically moved when undisturbed but stopped its movement when a dog was brought into the room. IBS symptoms including abdominal discomfort or pain, bloating and fullness, burning, constipation, and diarrhea have long been known to be associated with hyper- or hypoarousal of the autonomic nervous system.

The premise of this book is that there is a self-feeding sore-irritated tissue, leading to reflex guarding, anxiety, pain, and more guarding. We suggest here that this cycle may also be at work in IBS where chronic tightening of the colon leads to tissue irritation in the colon, leading to colonic spasm, pain, and protective guarding/spasm. In other words, we are suggesting that a set of cases of IBS may result from anxiety triggering colonic spasm, reflex guarding/spasm leading to anxiety, pain, and reflex guarding. The *Wise-Anderson Protocol* intervention we are suggesting, which is a modified form of the *Wise-Anderson Protocol,* may help break this tension-anxiety-pain cycle in IBS.

Irritable bowel syndrome, like chronic muscle-based pelvic pain, can be seen as a self-feeding cycle of irritated colonic tissue resulting from chronic colonic guarding promoted by anxiety, pain, protective guarding, and continued colonic irritation.

The simplicity and cost-effectiveness of this methodology are obvious. No drugs are used. Patients are empowered to help themselves. The risks are minimal. We are not proposing that readers of this book use these proposed methods for constipation, anal fissures, hemorrhoids, or irritable bowel syndrome without medical supervision, but we continue to endorse an experimental evaluation of this method for the symptoms of these related disorders.

Post–Bowel Movement Pain

One distressing symptom of pelvic pain occurs when a bowel movement flares it up. Little is written about this symptom when it occurs in the absence of hemorrhoids or anal fissures, but in our experience it is common.

In this section, we wish to propose an explanation of the mechanism responsible for this symptom and an intervention for it. The mechanism of defecation typically involves the filling up of the rectum with stool, which then sends a signal for the internal anal sphincter and puborectalis muscle to relax and triggers the experience of urgency to have a bowel movement. Once the stool passes through the relaxed anal sphincter and out of the body, the internal anal sphincter reflexively closes.

We propose that when someone has pelvic pain and exacerbation of symptoms after a bowel movement the internal anal sphincter tends to "overclose." That is, it tightens up more than it was tight before the bowel movement and sometimes appears to go into a kind of painful spasm. This, we suggest, is why some people have increased pain after a bowel movement.

> *Post–bowel movement discomfort usually occurs because the anal sphincter overcloses in a kind of spasm after a bowel movement in someone who has a chronically tightened pelvic basin.*

Our patients with post–bowel movement pain often insert a gloved, lubricated finger into the anal sphincter after a bowel movement to help release the overtightened sphincter. This maneuver can reduce post–bowel movement pain and sometimes can reduce or eliminate its appearance over time.

Post–bowel movement pain appears to occur less frequently when someone is relaxed and not hurried, and whatever contributes to a more relaxed state during a visit to the bathroom may reduce this symptom. The toilet manufacturer Toto makes a warm toilet seat called a Washlet that sends a warm stream of water, then air, to clean the anal opening after a bowel movement. This kind of post–bowel movement care may also be helpful for this symptom.

CHAPTER 6

PELVIC PAIN IN WOMEN

OUR PROTOCOL IS EQUALLY EFFECTIVE WITH WOMEN AND MEN IN OUR PUBLISHED STUDY

Muscle-based pelvic pain is not different in women than it is in men. In our 2016 study published in the journal *Applied Psychophysiology and Biofeedback,* Equal Improvement in Men and Women in the Treatment of Urologic Chronic Pelvic Pain Syndrome Using a Multi-modal Protocol with an Internal Myofascial Trigger Point Wand," we demonstrated that we have been able to help men and women equally with our protocol.

The treatment we use to help men or women is essentially the same. We have been able to help the same number of women as we help men with muscle-based pelvic pain using the *Wise-Anderson Protocol.* But there are conditions that affect only women, and we are gathering our insights into these various conditions in this chapter, both their causes and our insights about how to treat them.

We regularly evaluate and treat women diagnosed with conditions such as *interstitial cystitis (IC), urethral syndrome, painful bladder syndrome, pelvic floor dysfunction, levator ani syndrome, pelvic floor myalgia, dyspareunia, vulvodynia,* and *chronic pelvic pain,* among other diagnoses.

Women with pelvic pain often complain of one or more of the following kinds of symptoms (very few women have all symptoms):
- vaginal pain
- rectal pain
- pain around or above the pubic bone
- discomfort with sitting
- discomfort or pain with intercourse or sexual activity
- exacerbation of pelvic pain related to menstruation
- exacerbation of symptoms with stress and anxiety
- urinary frequency
- urinary urgency or hesitancy
- pain during or after urination
- pain during or after bowel movements
- pain related to childbirth

INTERSTITIAL CYSTITIS OR BLADDER PAIN SYNDROME

A majority of women who have participated in our program for pelvic pain have been diagnosed with the disorder of interstitial cystitis or bladder pain syndrome (IC/BPS). From epidemiological studies the prevalence of IC is estimated to be three hundred cases per one hundred thousand women. While men also have this condition, it is five to ten times more prevalent in women. IC is a chronic disease of unknown cause that is characterized by pelvic pain in multiple sites and bladder dysfunction, including urinary frequency and urgency, nocturia (desire to urinate during the night), and increased symptoms of urinary urgency with intercourse. Patients with IC may have only bladder symptoms and no other pain. While suprapubic pain or pain felt above the pubic bone is a prominent feature, additional pain sites include the urethra and genitalia, as well as others such as the groin, low back, thighs, and buttocks. This condition may coexist with other disorders, such as irritable bowel syndrome, fibromyalgia, vulvodynia, vulvar vestibulitis, pelvic floor dysfunction, Raynaud's syndrome, and migraine headache, among others.

Recently an international consortium of scientific experts met and voted to use the new term *bladder pain syndrome (BPS)* for the disorder commonly called interstitial cystitis or painful bladder syndrome. BPS is a clinical diagnosis encompassing the pattern of multiple symptoms as described above. For our discussions here we retain the IC terminology, although *IC* focuses narrowly on inflammation within the wall of the bladder and may not accurately describe the majority of patients with the syndrome. The trend at the present time is to identify the characteristics or phenotypes of chronic pelvic pain syndrome in women. Analyzing these categories may help narrow the focus of treatment.

The purpose of this chapter is to present a more comprehensive understanding of IC. We cannot provide all of the research on the condition or consider all theories but do include those approaches that best correspond to our experience in treating patients with IC. It is important to understand that IC remains a controversial diagnosis. Many clinicians think that it is a catchall diagnosis, a diagnosis of exclusion, and that its existence is not well substantiated, while others feel strongly that it is a definite condition with demonstrable pathology.

DESCRIPTIONS OF PAIN ASSOCIATED WITH INTERSTITIAL CYSTITIS

In a recent survey of 264 women with IC conducted by physicians at the University of Maryland and Johns Hopkins University, it was found that the respondents were quite precise in identifying multiple sites of pain, with pain sensations described as "throbbing, tender, piercing or aching." For genital pain sites, *burning, stinging,* and *sharp* were the pain descriptions. The most frequently reported sites of pain were the suprapubic, urethral, and genital areas, followed by other, nongenitourinary sites. Suprapubic and urethral pain were reported as worsening either with bladder filling or just before urination in 50 percent or more of the women. Approximately 80 percent of survey respondents also indicated pain worsening in these areas after consumption of certain food and drinks.

THEORIES TO EXPLAIN INTERSTITIAL CYSTITIS

IC may arise from a triggering event. A patient may have experienced a urinary infection, surgery, childbirth, a viral illness, or a physical or psychological trauma. Sensations of bladder pain then become a prominent feature. There is some evidence, as espoused by Dr. Tony Buffington, that an imbalance between the cortisone-producing endocrine system and a hyperactivated nervous system is responsible for the disorder. However, considerably more research is required to sort out the complexities involved.

One theory is that IC is a result of a neurovascular insult and that the symptoms of pain and urinary dysfunction are secondary to an ongoing process affecting the bladder. Drs. P. P. Irwin and Niall Galloway at Emory University have treated many patients with painful bladder disorders by blocking nerves in the lumbar area of the spinal cord to stop the natural adrenaline-producing nerve activity in the bladder.

There is evidence to suggest that IC may be due to overstimulation of the nerves to muscles and blood vessels in the bladder, which then results in spasm of the vessels and deprivation of oxygen to the organ.

This phenomenon of overstimulation has been shown to cause capillary blood vessel fragility in other parts of the body. The nerve blockade treatment that Erwin and Galloway employed temporarily improved the pain in many patients.

Physicians understand IC/BPS to be pelvic pain associated with urinary urgency and frequency. However, many women are incorrectly diagnosed as having a urinary tract infection (UTI), much as men are misdiagnosed as having chronic bacterial prostatitis, and thus are treated with a myriad of antimicrobial agents. Ironically, many women drink copious amounts of cranberry juice because it is thought to benefit a UTI, but cranberry juice actually may irritate IC symptoms. Some clinicians believe that the old diagnosis of urethral syndrome, associated with symptoms of urinary urgency, frequency, dysuria, suprapubic or low back pain, and voiding difficulties may be related to bladder pain syndrome.

DIAGNOSIS OF IC

A common diagnostic procedure for IC involves cystoscopy under anesthesia with bladder hydrodistension. The bladder is like a collapsed balloon when empty. The cystoscopic procedure involves filling the bladder with water to full capacity at relatively high pressure, then visualizing the wall of the bladder and the underlying blood vessels with a minicamera attached to a catheter inserted through the urethra into the bladder. A bladder that appears inflamed or even ulcerated and has small capillary vessel bleeding is thought to be indicative of IC. The bleeding results from fragility of blood vessels when the bladder is stretched. As the bladder is emptied, the tiny vessels rupture, creating small microhemorrhages and formation of a characteristic bloody pattern in the surface of the bladder.

The relevancy of some diagnostic tests for IC has been challenged. An example of this is cystoscopy under anesthesia with hydrodistension of the bladder. Some critics say that if you stretch anyone's bladder strongly enough, you can probably make it bleed. However, the diagnostic test is meaningful only if the patient has all the rest of the hallmarks of chronic pelvic pain and urinary symptoms.

Bladder distension (stretching) under anesthesia is also currently used as a therapeutic tool to manage IC. About 30 percent of patients, a relatively small and unimpressive proportion, note a sustained improvement after undergoing this procedure. Biopsy of the bladder is rarely necessary as no serious diseases are uncovered, although superficial bladder cancer needs to be ruled out.

One finding related to IC is that the mucosal lining of the bladder, known as the glycosaminoglycan (GAG) layer, may not be providing an adequate barrier function for the bladder. Defects in the integrity of the GAG layer may allow micropores or tiny gaps in the mucosa to develop, allowing urinary metabolites or toxins, especially potassium, to penetrate the lining through to the submucosal receptors of nerves and blood vessels. When a physician introduces potassium solutions into the bladder of someone suffering from IC, this causes pain, and some believe that this observation serves to confirm the leakage of noxious stimuli into the submucosa layer of the bladder. This commonly used diagnostic test for IC aims to determine whether the potassium solution causes more pain than water when introduced into the bladder. One of the questions about this test is whether there is any association between the sensitivity of the bladder to potassium and the finding of the blood vessel fragility on stretching of the bladder. Dr. Mireille Grégoire from Quebec showed no difference in blood vessel fragility in those who had positive potassium tests and those who did not. The merit of the potassium test as a diagnostic indicator for IC may be called into question.

Neurogenic Inflammation in the Bladder

IC is a bladder condition generally involving inflammation. Dr. Ragi Doggweiler and others have discussed the theory of neurogenic inflammation as it relates to the bladder. This theory is compelling. Neurogenic inflammation is an inflammatory process that is induced through stimulation of nerve receptors.

In the model of neurogenic inflammation, an insult to the bladder or pelvic floor may send messages to the part of the spine that controls bladder and pelvic floor function, causing "neural windup" and a cascade of events resulting in inflammation.

In this conceptual model of neurogenic inflammation, an insult to the bladder or pelvic floor, which may be physical, such as postdelivery trauma or frequent urinary tract infections, or a psychological stressor, such as intense anxiety or physical stress, may be an initiating factor in the development of IC symptoms. This stressful perpetrator in the bladder and pelvic floor is thought to send messages to the part of the spine that controls bladder and pelvic floor function. These intense signals to the spinal cord from the pelvic muscles produce what is called *neural windup,* in which the activity of the nervous system in the spine becomes strongly aroused.

The Wise-Anderson Protocol *attempts*
to break the cycle of neural windup.

This windup of the activity in the spinal nerves (initiated from signals from the pelvis) is thought to cause a high level of nervous activity in the pelvis and bladder. The neural windup is believed to create a cascade of events that results in inflammation. In this neural windup model, we have a self-feeding cycle of increased pain and increased anxiety, which continues to support the arousal and the windup of the nervous system. This then supports inflammation, causing more pain and contraction, which lead to more inflammation and anxiety. This is a difficult cycle to break. The *Wise-Anderson Protocol* described in this book attempts to intervene in this cycle.

Anxiety and Interstitial Cystitis

Madlen Oemler and associates in Germany reported that people with IC had a higher level of life adversity than normal subjects without IC (controls), on the basis of a survey of accumulative childhood experiences. Survey results revealed that IC patients tended to have a poor emotional relationship with their parents, a more difficult and anxiety-laden childhood, and indications of physical abuse. IC patients had higher scores for dysfunction than the controls.

Numerous studies have shown that stress and anxiety impair the healing of wounds. Elizabeth Broadbent and coworkers in New Zealand recently reported that psychological stress is associated with slower wound healing. They suggested that reduction of psychological stress can improve wound repair following surgery. Christos Pitsavos and his team in Greece showed that anxiety increases inflammation in healthy people. In Sweden, Annsofi Johanssen and colleagues found a positive relationship between the occurrence of gum inflammation and anxiety.

Giorgio Grossi and his team in Sweden found that stress in women tends to result in increased inflammation. In Israel, Samuel Melamed and colleagues found that the fear of terrorism promoted increased levels of low-grade inflammation in apparently healthy adults. Il Song and his team in British Columbia reported that increased anxiety and stress produced an inflammatory response in laboratory rats. Lin Ying Liu and associates in Wisconsin found that anxiety during examination taking exacerbated the inflammatory response in asthma.

Anxiety is a proinflammatory state.

Although it appears that anxiety is proinflammatory and interferes with the body's natural healing mechanisms, there is little current evidence on the effect of lowering anxiety and general nervous system arousal and the improvement of IC.

Anxiety and Mucous Membrane Inflammation, a Common Denominator for Many Syndromes

The bladder is lined with mucosa (a mucous membrane). In this section we will discuss the similar effects of anxiety on inflammation of the mucosa in other body areas in order to gain insight about inflammation and the bladder.

Mucosa lines all the cavities of the body that open externally, including the nose, mouth, esophagus, stomach, intestines, bladder, vagina, and lungs. Inflammation, ulceration, and pain can occur in all body locations lined with mucous membranes. Anxiety has been associated with onset and exacerbation of inflammation in mucosal tissues. Thus the strong effect of anxiety on bladder conditions is not unexpected, nor should reduced anxiety be unexpected to have an equally powerful healing effect.

Stewart Wolf and Harold G. Wolff found that "sustained hyper function" of the bowel was associated with increased fragility of the bowel's mucous membrane in such a way that even minor stresses resulted in hemorrhage or ulceration. This was particularly evident in individuals with ulcerative colitis. While these patients appeared outwardly calm and superficially peaceful, underneath this apparent placid demeanor the person often sat on "a powder keg" of intense hostility, resentment, and guilt. These long-standing, unrelieved feelings were associated with hyperfunction of the colon with increased motor activity, increased vascularity, turgescence, and small hemorrhagic lesions.

Anxiety appears to promote gum inflammation.

If you speak to dentists, they will tell you that patients who are anxious or significantly stressed often have gums that are puffy and inflamed. This observation is supported by the research of Johanssen in Sweden and Mario Vianna Vettore in Brazil, which indicates the adverse effect of anxiety on gum inflammation.

Irritable bowel syndrome, a very common condition of pain, bloating, and disturbed bowel habits, is associated with mucosal inflammation. Numerous studies support the association between anxiety and bowel mucosal inflammation. Wolf and Wolff in their classic book *The Colon* documented the change in color and mucous secretion of subjects who became anxious or agitated.

Inflammation of the esophagus mucosa, called gastroesophageal reflux disorder (GERD—or more commonly heartburn) and esophagitis (inflammation of the esophagus), nausea, functional idiopathic dyspepsia, gastritis, stomach ulceration, burning mouth syndrome, and even anal fissures are associated with anxiety.

DEPRESSIVE SYMPTOMS AND QUALITY OF LIFE IN INTERSTITIAL CYSTITIS PATIENTS

A recent publication by Dr. Nan Rothrock of the University of Iowa indicates that IC patients have poor functioning in various life domains and that with increased severity of symptoms there is further deterioration in quality of life.

It is always difficult for physicians, friends,
and acquaintances to appreciate the
extent of disability and suffering resulting
from a chronic pelvic pain disorder.

IC adversely affects leisure activities, family relations, and travel in 70 to 94 percent of patients. Depression and fatigue are common experiences for these patients, as are difficulty concentrating and insomnia. The University of Iowa study involved only IC female patients who completed questionnaires for psychological assessment, including depressive symptoms. Bladder biopsies also were examined. A comparative control group of forty age-matched women without IC completed the depression questionnaires. The study showed that the IC patients with more severe disease had significantly greater limitations in their physical and social functioning, as well as a greater impact on their mental health. Of interest is that bladder biopsies revealed the absence of only mild inflammation in 80 percent of the patients and no ulceration in 80 percent. However, 80 percent of patients had moderate to severe capillary fragility with petechial hemorrhages (pinpoint bleeding). No specific IC symptom was associated with depression. The positive note in this study is that although IC patients had proportionally more depression than healthy controls, there was very little severe depression, and patients were able to cope with their normal life experiences.

INTERVENING IN THE POSSIBLE SELF-FEEDING CYCLE OF IC

The constellation of pelvic trauma, chronic pelvic pain, protective guarding against pain, chronic pelvic tension including pain-referring trigger points, and a predisposition toward anxiety and catastrophic thinking that feeds anxiety and inflammation in the bladder may all be part of a self-feeding, self-perpetuating cycle in women and men with IC. As with male pelvic pain, the goal of our *Wise-Anderson Protocol* is to interrupt this cascade of events.

*Anxiety is almost always significantly
reduced in IC patients when they feel they
can do something to help themselves.*

In our view, quieting nervous system arousal needs to be done regularly, especially because IC patients may have a greater predisposition toward anxiety or have relatively more anxiety as a result of their condition. While patients may become discouraged when hearing this, we are not: we simply feel that it takes more effort and intention to reduce the general level of nervousness in order for patients to help themselves. Quieting anxiety in our protocol includes both regular practice in inducing profound relaxation, managing thinking that tends to spin off into catastrophic imaginings, and dealing with lifestyle issues and one's relationships.

TRIGGER POINTS AND IC

*Typically a large number of trigger points
are found in those diagnosed with IC.*

We have found that individuals with IC often have a large number of trigger points in the pelvic floor that are often very painful. These trigger points can be accessed and manipulated by a physical therapist. However, we strongly believe that it is important that IC patients also be taught how to identify and work on the trigger points themselves.

RESEARCH ON DIET AND IC

In IC, unlike other conditions of pelvic pain where there is no clear association with foods that may induce symptoms, the management of one's diet may be important. If one continually eats foods and drinks beverages that irritate the bladder, this practice will undermine other aspects of treatment. Physicians have suggested caffeine, alcohol, spicy, acidic, or tomato-containing foods, carbonated drinks, and even multi-vitamins as possible aggravating factors for IC. Many patients can identify other foods that presumably create difficulty.

However, strict dietary directives may not be useful and are often unnecessarily restrictive. It makes sense to eliminate foods only if one knows they will affect one's bladder because painful bladder symptoms occur. An ongoing evaluation is useful, as sensitivities to specific foods may vary from time to time. We strongly suggest keeping a diary to identify the food or drinks that appear to be associated with subsequent increased pain or urinary frequency and urgency.

In a recent study, Robert Moldwin, Barbara Shorter, and colleagues at Long Island University examined the effect of foods, beverages, and supplements on IC patients. Study results suggested that elimination of coffee, tea, alcoholic beverages, citrus fruits and juices, spicy foods, hot peppers, and certain artificial sweeteners may have a positive effect on reducing a patient's symptoms. This is in agreement with much of the conventional wisdom among IC patient advocate groups. However, some studies have found little difference in ingesting substances that alkalinize the urine. In general, monitoring of diet probably has a role in controlling IC symptoms, but elimination of possibly offending foods has not been shown to be curative.

CURRENT MANAGEMENT AND TREATMENT OF IC

Several therapeutic approaches are currently being used to manage the symptoms of IC. These include oral medications, injection of agents directly into the bladder lining, and instillations of agents into the bladder through a catheter.

Several pharmaceutical drugs have been used to manage IC symptoms. Only one oral drug is approved by the US Food and Drug Administration (FDA) for the specific indication of IC. However, its usefulness is questionable. Pentosan polysulfate sodium (Elmiron) is intended to improve the GAG layer of the bladder. In multiple clinical trials of this drug,

28 to 40 percent of all patients were reported to have had significant improvement. The drug must be used for an extended period of three to six months to achieve the greatest benefit. In an NIH-sponsored clinical trial, the effects of Elmiron, and the antihistamine called hydroxyzine used as single agents or in combination and compared with a placebo were evaluated. Thirty-four percent of patients had a response (reduction of symptoms) with Elmiron compared with 18 percent of patients on placebo. With the antihistamine alone, 31 percent of patients had a response, as did 20 percent on placebo. When both drugs were taken together, 40 percent of patients obtained a response.

The overall conclusion was that neither of the
drugs, either used alone or in combination,
resulted in significant enough improvement
of IC symptoms to warrant further study.

It is a consensus of the NIH research groups that amitriptyline (Elavil), a long-term traditional antidepressant, might be beneficial in reducing painful bladder syndrome. National trials are under way to determine the effectiveness of this agent versus placebo.

Instillation of drugs into the bladder such as steroids, anesthetics, and antibiotic solutions are treatment approaches to ease pain and frequency in IC patients. Dimethyl sulfoxide (DMSO) has been approved for this purpose, and reports have indicated that up to 70 percent of IC patients experience some relief of symptoms. Often physicians will create a "cocktail" with DMSO, adding hydrocortisone, alkalinizing sodium bicarbonate, lidocaine or Marcaine (a topical anesthetic), and heparin to act as a surface sealant. Initially there also was hope that immune modulation of the bladder surface by instillation of a tuberculosis vaccine (BCG) would provide some benefit for IC. However, when this approach was tested against a placebo in national clinical trials no meaningful benefit was achieved. Hyaluronic acid (Cystistat) has not been approved in the United States, but reports of benefit after placement in the bladder have come from Canadian studies.

Approximately 5 to 10 percent of patients with IC have lesions called

Hunner's ulcers on the bladder wall. Removing the ulcers with fulguration, "burning" them off with electrical cautery or laser treatment, or excising the lesion and surrounding tissue can bring relief. The ulcers can reoccur, and repeat treatment is recommended when symptoms reappear. A new treatment under evaluation involves injection of a steroid. Some patients just live with their ulcers, and some attempt to gain symptom relief by removing acidic food and drinks from their diet, if indeed these appear to aggravate their condition.

Bladder conditioning, namely stretching the bladder with timed voiding, is a nonpharmacological and patient-directed approach. This conditioning helps to desensitize IC patients to the sensation of needing to void. They are taught to gradually stretch the bladder by deferring urination for several minutes each day, attempting to increase the total volume voided. It is important to do this throughout the day with increased fluid intake and to void by the clock rather than succumb to the urgency they feel. When needed, we teach techniques to suppress the urgency. However, if patients' discomfort is more than 6 or 7 on a scale of 10, then they need to give in to the urge to urinate.

*Pelvic floor physical therapy has been
shown in some studies to be very helpful
for those diagnosed with IC.*

Reduction of pelvic floor muscle irritation and hypertonicity and bladder-related trigger points, usually benefits this group of patients. In a California study, Jerome Weiss reported that treatment of urgency/frequency syndrome with intrapelvic myofascial release treatment resulted in reduced symptoms. The study involved both men and women. Of the forty-two patients who had urgency/frequency (with or without pain) for six to fourteen years, 83 percent had moderate to marked improvement or complete resolution. Weiss postulated that the bladder is not completely responsible for the symptoms and that the pelvic floor and the sphincter muscles play a major role. These patients typically have tender spots in the pelvis on palpation, a finding consistent with the trigger points we have described. Many patients with the diagnosis of IC describe difficult voiding in childhood and may have had previous trauma contributing to their dysfunction, even triggering events that appear so trivial as to not be recognized as a cause.

Anatomically the pelvic floor myofascial trigger points may influence the bladder. This occurs because their nerve nuclei or origins lie in close proximity within the spinal cord to incoming nerve endings from bladder autonomic nerves. Flare-ups of IC, including pain and urinary urgency, can be activated by stress, dietary indiscretions, improper exercise or movement, trauma, sexual activity, cold weather, hormonal shifts, and viral infection. Details of the actual neurophysiologic changes within the nervous system and within the muscular tissue have yet to be worked out by the basic scientists, but clinicians continue to seek the relationships that may guide basic investigation.

A recent national clinical trial utilizing manual pelvic physical therapy to treat eighty-one women with IC at eleven different centers *showed 59 percent of them improving to a moderate or markedly improved status.*

POTENTIAL THERAPEUTIC APPROACHES FOR IC UNDER EVALUATION

Attention is being drawn to the potential of gene therapy for IC bladder pain. While it is in the early stages of research in animal bladders, scientists are using the herpes simplex virus as a "carrier" for a gene for a substance that participates in the synthesis of a natural painkiller in the body. When animals with bladder irritation got the gene, there was lower bladder hyperactivity and less pain-related behavior. Laboratory analysis showed that the gene had been incorporated into the bladder and the nerve roots that receive pain impulses from the bladder.

Researchers are exploring new drug targets to ease bladder pain and hypersensitivity. They are focusing on receptors or protein molecules embedded in the outside surface (plasma membrane) or within cells (the cytoplasm). Drugs can be designed to bind to the receptors and specifically block processes that excite bladder activity. One such experimental agent blocks a prostaglandin receptor in the central nervous system and may help control bladder overactivity and pain. Another drug targets spinal corticotropin-releasing factor (CRF), which is released when animals are stressed, resulting in hypersensitivity to pain. This last study supports the role of stress in making bladder pain worse and implicates spinal cord CRF-like compounds and their receptors in the process. Yet another approach is targeting the sensory nerves in the bladder and their receptors. When ATP (adenosine triphosphate), a major source of energy for cellular reactions, or similar compounds attach to the nerve receptors they become more sensitive to noxious or irritating stimulation. Blocking of the ATP receptors fully blocked certain types of chronic inflammation and neuropathic pain.

Another innovative and experimental approach utilizes forms of electrical stimulation for symptom relief in patients with IC. In a process similar to acupuncture, the electrical pulses are targeted to nerves that send signals from the pelvis to the spinal cord. Electrode leads may be implanted into the sacral nerves, near the pudendal nerve or the tibial nerve in the ankle. The more common therapy involves sacral neuromodulation to alleviate overactive bladder. Pudendal nerve stimulation has been used when sacral stimulation stops working or does not work. Dr. Ken Peters and colleagues at William Beaumont Hospital in Michigan recently treated a group of patients, most with prior sacral neuromodulation; 71 percent of the eighty-four patients had 50 percent symptom improvements described as significant for frequency, voided volume, incontinence, and urgency. Some of the patients had complications, requiring revisions in seven and reoperations in four others. The effectiveness of electrical nerve stimulation of the tibial nerve near the ankle has been compared with extended release tolterodine (Detrol LA) for treatment of overactive bladder. While objective measurements showed similar improvements in both groups, more patients who got the nerve stimulation said they were cured or improved than those on the drug. These nerve stimulation procedures have been approved by the FDA for treatment of overactive bladder; they may have potential in IC but have not been specifically evaluated or approved for pain relief in patients with IC.

VULVODYNIA

Vulvodynia or hypersensitivity of the vulva and vaginal opening was first described in the nineteenth century. It includes disorders named *vulvar vestibulitis* and *essential vulvodynia*. The incidence and prevalence of these conditions are not definitively known. Some estimates suggest that up to 15 percent of women with IC also have vulvar pain. Typically 50 percent of women with vulvodynia experience dyspareunia, which is pain during or right after sexual intercourse. They feel pain during penile insertion into the vagina, as well as pain while inserting tampons. *Vulvar vestibulitis* is defined as inflammation of the tissue at the vaginal entrance with a pronounced redness and exquisite sensitivity when touched even lightly. Sharp pain occurs when this delicate skin is rubbed, and this pain often prohibits or limits normal sexual intercourse. Even clothing such as pantyhose or tight-fitting lingerie may be irritating.

This disorder commonly occurs in sexually active young women and can even develop after previous normal, nonpainful sexual intercourse. It is not unusual for these women to have a coincident occurrence of IC with their vulvodynia. Many women are misdiagnosed as having fungal vaginitis, lichen planus, or contact dermatitis and are treated with antifungal agents and other topical medications; these may even worsen some of the inflammatory responses. Some have suggested there is coinciding subclinical infection of the human papilloma virus or genital wart virus, but there is no scientific proof.

Patients are frequently treated with medications such as antidepressants (e.g., Elavil) for neuropathic pain, topical estrogens, and cortisone creams.

Surgical or destructive manipulations of the
tissues typically have a disappointing outcome.

PELVIC PAIN AND MENSTRUATION

Today girls are reaching menarche at younger ages. The extreme pain and spasm experienced by some very young women before and during their menstrual flow may be related to the tightness developed in their pelvises because of earlier conditioning. Normalizing pelvic muscle tone and function or even simply adding an aerobic component to one's exercise program is sometimes helpful for a more comfortable menses.

PELVIC PAIN AND PREGNANCY

Hormonal changes during pregnancy cause a softening of connective tissue. Poor posture, slouching, or sitting with pressure on the coccyx (tailbone) could predispose it to strain and pain. This is an ideal time to learn to sit without pressure on the coccyx. Ideally, sitting erect with a normal concave curve in the lumbar spine and transmitting weight through the ischial tuberosities (sitting bones at the bottom of the pelvis) may go a long way in preventing coccydynia/coccygodynia (tailbone pain) during the childbearing years. Once this condition develops, it may be necessary to sit on a cushion to reduce pressure on the coccyx, thereby transmitting weight through the thighs and ischial tuberosities.

ROUND LIGAMENT PAIN

Round ligament pain sometimes occurs in pregnant women. It is a sharp stitch-like pain in the lower abdomen and groin, often lasting up to twenty minutes and caused by sudden changes in posture, such as rolling over in bed or standing from a sitting position. The round ligaments are fibromuscular cords that help support the uterus and extend into the labia majora. These ligaments can become hypertrophied or enlarged and more vascular during pregnancy to support the increased weight of the baby. Gently pulling in the belly and tilting the pelvis backwards to support the baby before changing position is sometimes suggested to help this problem. Occasionally a support belt may be useful with a large baby or multiple pregnancies.

URINARY URGENCY AND FREQUENCY DURING PREGNANCY

Urinary urgency and frequency can occur as normal sensations during early and late pregnancy. In the first trimester, the uterus becomes heavier and presses on the bladder and does not allow it to expand as usual. In the last trimester, the pressure of the baby's head moving into position for birth often makes a woman feel a constant urgency to urinate.

SYMPHYSIS PUBIS PAIN AND PREGNANCY

This is also caused by ligamentous laxity during pregnancy, which causes increased movement of the joint holding the pelvis together in front. Avoiding unilateral weight bearing or exercise, wearing a sacroiliac belt, and consulting with a physical therapist for stabilizing postural exercise and activities of daily living can be helpful.

DIASTASIS OF THE RECTUS ABDOMINIS

What is referred to as the belly of the rectus abdominis muscles tends to separate during pregnancy because of both hormonal and anatomical changes. Since the abdominal muscles play a key role in posture and good body mechanics (which directly relate to pelvic pain), it is important to be aware of ways of minimizing muscle separation during any exercise program.

PELVIC PAIN FROM LABOR AND DELIVERY

The physical efforts of labor and delivery can greatly affect a woman's pelvic floor and can set the stage for a number of pelvic pain syndromes. Even in ideal birthing situations, the pelvic floor muscles can stretch up to one and a half times their normal length, sometimes resulting in overstretched nerves or even rupture of some muscle fibers.

In Western civilizations, birthing women are predisposed to other problems as well. In collaboration with health care providers, couples are more prone to request induction of labor for their convenience instead of allowing nature to take its course. Rupturing of membranes artificially or use of hormones like Pitocin to speed up the labor process can make labor and delivery much more painful and difficult for a woman. This often necessitates the use of more pain medications, a resultant loss of control, and the need for larger episiotomies and even instrumentation. A gentler, more natural process, even if longer, is kinder to the pelvic floor. Of course, some conditions necessitate intervention for the health of the baby or mother; choosing an obstetrician sensitive to these issues is important.

*Labor and delivery can sometimes trigger
certain pelvic pain syndromes.*

Birthing in more difficult antigravity positions is unfortunately still common, as are the use of analgesic or anesthetic agents that decrease or nullify active labor and delivery participation by the mother. Instrumentation in the form of forceps delivery, when employed, sometimes results in large episiotomies and tears.

Unfortunately, it is not unusual to hear some women complain of pelvic pain or dysfunction after childbirth. Pain or dysfunction persisting for six weeks or more after delivery necessitates professional care. Most complaints are of weakness, stress, or urinary or bowel incontinence. A program of graduated pelvic floor exercise and behavioral training is usually sufficient to correct these problems. However, dyspareunia (pain during and/or after intercourse) or difficulty and pain during or right after a bowel movement can be the result of poor healing or scar tissue formation and, rarely, even the vaginal opening being too tightly sutured during episiotomy repair.

With a very large baby or a difficult presentation like posterior, face, or breech, the pelvic bones sometimes separate, especially if instrumentation like forceps or suction is used. The mother may have pain or may not be able to turn over in bed or get up to walk. She also may have vaginal, suprapubic, sacroiliac, and groin pain. Bowel movements may increase her pain, and urinary pain, urgency, and frequency are often present. A timely rehabilitation is possible with a disciplined program of non-weight-bearing pelvic stabilization with a belt and appropriate exercise combined with myofascial release and trigger point release. However, this can be a difficult task for a new mother. Occasionally, injections into the pubic symphysis and sacroiliac joints are necessary to enhance stability (prolo-therapy).

REDUCING THE RISK OF PELVIC PAIN AFTER CHILDBIRTH

Conventional wisdom is not always wise. The conventional wisdom in the past endorsed midline episiotomies and turned an indifferent eye to prolonged second-stage labor and to large weight gain during pregnancy, among other practices. But the obstetrical understanding with regard to childbirth has changed in recent years. Below are some important considerations when making plans about childbirth. These are even more important if there is an existing pelvic pain condition.

> *The philosophy guiding childbirth may profoundly affect the woman's experience and her chances of developing pelvic pain.*

The facility chosen in which to give birth is an important decision, particularly in terms of its having a sympathetic gentle birthing philosophy and methodology. A relaxed birthing atmosphere that is as homelike and comfortable as possible is important because it enables the laboring mother to be more relaxed and at ease.

We also consider it important to choose a health professional empathetic to the ideals of natural gentle birthing. This could be a midwife or physician who is comfortable with a woman laboring and delivering in different positions—someone who sincerely endorses this and is not simply giving lip service to these ideas but is committed to and has had experience in the practice of them.

Obviously there is a place for medical monitors and intravenous drips in difficult or complicated deliveries. However, in the absence of the need for monitoring and medical intervention, we think it important that a woman be free to walk around, get down on all fours and gently rock, rhythmically "dance," moving her pelvis from side to side (there are reports that belly dancing originated as a childbirth ritual), or bounce gently on a big birthing ball. A birthing ball is a large, sturdy, inflatable ball that a mother sits on and can rhythmically bounce on. It is sometimes recommended in order for a mother to help her baby to find the best position to travel down through the pelvis and birth canal.

The subject of birthing is far beyond the scope of this book. Suffice it to say that we prefer natural birthing in as homelike an environment as possible. This is in contrast to turning birthing mothers into hospital patients and transforming a beautiful and natural human process into a medical procedure.

Many birthing experts support an expectant
mother staying at home as long as possible.

A good childbirth educator and/or *doula* (a specially trained labor assistant) may be consulted to help with the decision of when, during the final stages of labor, to go to the birthing facility. The importance of staying as long as possible in a comfortable and stress-free environment is illustrated in studies on mice. When the birthing environment of mice is disturbed, by gently lifting the laboring mother and placing her in another location, her delivery is significantly delayed, the equivalent of many hours in a human being.

It is recommended to find the most experienced childbirth educator available. Someone in private practice may feel freer to teach you about all the choices available. A hospital, or a physician-employed educator of the hospital, may be more likely to direct you toward their facility. Some have said that employing the services of a *doula* who can navigate the system is a good investment. The *doula* usually has the time, patience, and physical and emotional skills needed to support a natural and mother-centered birthing experience. It is obviously important to get in good physical shape with a good exercise program that helps stretch the muscles necessary for birth and to train endurance, proper relaxation, and posture.

It is important to learn how to contract and especially how to release pelvic muscles to facilitate birthing. Daily massaging, warming the vaginal muscles, and stretching the vaginal opening with a natural oil like almond, sesame, or olive may be helpful to avoid tearing during childbirth. It is important to note that while we consider yoga to be helpful in preparation for childbirth, overly vigorous yoga can overstretch ligaments (which are already softened with the hormone relaxin). A yoga teacher who understands the kind of gentle stretching that is helpful for childbirth is essential. The second stage of childbirth has to do with the cervix dilating to about ten centimeters. The popular image of this stage is that of the soon-to-be mother, with cheering from others in the room, pushing hard for a long time to release the baby. There is more and more agreement, however, that strong, prolonged pushing during the second stage of childbirth is not a good idea. Gentle pushing is imperative as is a not-too-prolonged second stage of labor. If one has ever watched a calf or puppy being born, one will observe how the mother pants gently, pushes a little, and then goes back to panting. When a woman cooperates with her body, her uterus is usually able to do its work, and it is the uterus that does most of the work in expelling a baby.

Many natural birthing advocates consider a
mother's position at birth to be important.

Many women in third-world countries, who are used to squatting, typically give birth squatting. In a squatting position the pelvic outlet widens. Some birthing consultants report that when women are given the opportunity to choose any position during the second stage of labor, most will opt for being supported in a half squat. This way the birth is gravity assisted.

As we have mentioned, prolonged pushing and a prolonged second stage of labor are considered by many obstetricians a part of childbirth to be avoided, as this raises the risk of tissue tearing and postpartum pain and incontinence. Additionally, it can cause stretching of the nerves and muscles, which can result in weakness, pelvic prolapse, and incontinence (especially when hormonal changes during menopause occur).

Related to this is the current trend to avoid episiotomy, the cutting of the perineum to permit a wider opening for the exit of the child. Both mediolateral episiotomies, in which the cut is made laterally into the perineum, and medial episiotomies, in which the incision is straight down toward the perineum, are not recommended by many obstetricians, as these can facilitate a larger tear. Again, the exception is when the life of the child or the mother is at stake.

Weight control, stretching of the muscles related to childbirth, and practice in relaxation can make childbirth easier and can tend to reduce the risk of pelvic trauma and pelvic pain.

The case against episiotomy can be understood from experience in the fabric store. Typically, to more easily tear or cut a fabric, you make an initial small cut. In the same way, the episiotomy tends to facilitate more tearing in the tissue than the natural and spontaneous tearing that might occur during childbirth. A skilled professional is important at the birth to help make the appropriate decision about episiotomy, as a severely torn perineum or pelvic floor is a major problem and not easy to repair.

Also, contrary to the indifference of conventional wisdom with regard to weight gain, many obstetricians suggest to limit weight gain to not more than twenty to thirty pounds. More weight tends to mean bigger babies, which tends to mean more risk of trauma in getting them out.

Exercises that tighten the abdomen are often not friendly to easy childbirth. Some doctors report that dancers, for example, tend to have more difficulty in childbirth because their pelvis and abdomen have been trained to remain tight and constricted. What has emerged in recent times is that weight control, stretching, and relaxation techniques tend to make childbirth easier and diminish the likelihood of trauma.

Finally, relaxation has been universally appreciated in facilitating childbirth. In the same way as we support patients to not be afraid of pain and to relax with pain, so we need to support mothers giving birth to relax with discomfort and pain instead of contracting against it. The mother who has practiced appropriate stretching and relaxation even in the presence of discomfort has a better chance of an easier birth.

DYSPAREUNIA (PAINFUL INTERCOURSE)

Pain during intercourse can often be significantly reduced or eliminated if the chronic contraction of the pelvic floor is loosened and if internal pelvic floor trigger points and areas of restriction are released. This problem can manifest at a very young age when teenagers find that inserting even a small tampon during menstruation is too painful. These are often the same women who find it difficult to have a gynecological exam because insertion of a speculum into the vagina causes pain. Sometimes they are not even able to tolerate the physician's examining finger.

Mostly these problems stem from chronic muscle tightness or guarding, but there are instances where the hymen may be thicker than normal and can result in more of a physical barrier. Most patients respond well to vaginal massage and stretching, trigger point release, and pelvic floor relaxation. Rarely does this condition require surgery.

A young woman with dyspareunia came to see us after having had two children. Her marriage had never been consummated. Instead, she was artificially impregnated with her husband's sperm and had a cesarean birth for both children. In her midthirties, both she and her husband finally decided to confront her inability to have intercourse. After one consultation, where they were taught the techniques of vaginal massage and paradoxical relaxation, the couple was finally able to have sexual intercourse. Most often, however, more factors are involved in vaginismus (or spasm and tightness of the vaginal muscles), requiring more extensive myofascial release and trigger point release, as well as psychological and sex counseling.

VAGINISMUS

Vaginismus refers to a usually instantaneous, painful tightening/spasm of the muscles around the entrance of the vagina. The normal state of these vaginal muscles is closed. Typically when relaxed the vagina is able to open, allowing the woman to engage in sexual intercourse, the insertion of a tampon, or the insertion of a finger during a medical examination. This abrupt vaginal spasm can derive from experiences earlier in life relating to cultural conditioning, sexual trauma, or a negative sexual experience. Aside from being painful and usually out of the woman's control, it can profoundly affect a woman's life by interfering with the normal development of an intimate relationship, allowing her to be sexual or to bear children. It is a difficult situation for any woman to be physically unable to develop an intimate sexual relationship because of this condition.

The difference between someone with vaginismus and the pelvic pain that we have treated is that typically a woman with vaginismus has vaginal pain and constriction only in anticipation of or during sexual activity, medical examination, or tampon insertion. The *Wise-Anderson Protocol* is usually able to help a woman overcome this condition by teaching her to do her own trigger point release, paradoxical relaxation, and vaginal stretching, sometimes with graduated sizes of vaginal dilators.

The Wise-Anderson Protocol *has been able
to help selected women overcome vaginismus.*

In our view, vaginismus is not simply a physical problem of tight or spastic muscles; like many pelvic pain conditions, it may involve negative past conditioning and attitudes.

MENOPAUSE

As women approach menopause and hormone levels drop, less mucus is secreted and the vaginal tissue can become more fragile. Painful intercourse, urinary urgency, frequency, or even incontinence can attend this time of life. Estrogen replacement therapy (ERT) or local estrogen replacement inserted into the vaginal opening can be helpful. This augments vaginal tissue health and can even help with stress incontinence if the problem is mainly urethral tissue thinning. A program of pelvic floor muscle exercises, using both slow and fast contractions (even doing six five- to ten-second contractions followed by ten quick vaginal muscle flicks after each urination), can make a difference. This can be helpful in combination with vaginal stretching and gentle trigger point release and myofascial release and is often all that is necessary.

PELVIC PAIN IN A LARGER CONTEXT

It is easy to "medicalize" the subject of pelvic pain in general and women's pelvic pain in particular. In doing so, one can lose sight of the larger picture that *a woman who has pelvic pain is more than her pelvic pain*. In our view, other important factors are often involved in female pelvic pain aside from specific symptoms that conventional medicine takes into account. A woman's pelvic pain is present along with her anxiety and general level of nervous system arousal, her early conditioning, the quality of her relationships, her skill in relationships, and the level of her insight into her thinking, her emotions, and her past. Pelvic pain, as we understand it and describe it in this book, may be the consequence of, or may be exacerbated by, how some women (and men) express their fears and suppress their feelings in order to maintain equilibrium in their lives. In discussing this, we are not in any way negating the fact that there also may have been a provoking trauma or medical reason for the initiation of the pain syndrome.

EMOTIONS AND PELVIC PAIN: AN ILLUSTRATION

During the writing of the fourth edition of our book, a physical therapist with whom we work closely reported doing a session with a woman with pelvic pain who had experienced an intense flare-up of her symptoms after having a substantial period of being pain-free after practicing our protocol. She began seeing the therapist in an attempt to reverse the flare-up.

During the course of the physical therapy session a remarkable event occurred. It was remarkable not because it was uncommon (indeed, it is the most common of events) but because the event was witnessed in a therapeutic setting. This is what happened.

During the physical therapy session, while the therapist had her finger inside the patient's vagina, the patient began to talk about something about which she was very upset. As the woman shared her upset feelings, the therapist felt her finger being crushed in a vise-like grip of the woman's pelvic muscle contraction. The patient was middle-aged, and the physical therapist was amazed at the strength of contraction of the muscles of this woman's pelvic floor while she shared her upset feelings—a strength of contraction not even felt in the pelvic strength of substantially younger women.

"Did you feel that?" the physical therapist asked her patient. "Did I feel what?" replied the patient. "Can't you feel the spasm that your pelvis has gone into right now while you are talking about these upsetting things?" asked the physical therapist. The patient was dumbfounded. "I don't feel anything," replied the patient. She had no sense of the relationship between her emotions and the reaction of her pelvic muscles. Only after a number of attempts on the part of our colleague to help the patient re-create her upsetting feelings and simultaneously feel her pelvic muscles contract was the patient able to appreciate what was going on inside her pelvis when she was upset.

The pelvis, for those with pelvic pain, can be thought of as the site of their "gut reaction." Perhaps what could be called a gut reaction in some people could be called a pelvic reaction in those with pelvic pain. We believe that whenever someone with pelvic pain is upset or concerned, without any training to abort this, pelvic floor contraction is a component. This is particularly true when a pelvic floor is sore or hyperirritable and its contraction is set off by very small events that otherwise would have no effect on the person if the pelvis was not sore and irritated. Consequently our protocol emphasizes teaching patients the skill of profoundly relaxing their pelvic muscles and regularly lowering their level of anxiety.

CHAPTER 7

THE MEDICAL SCIENCE OF CHRONIC PELVIC PAIN

This chapter offers insight into what physicians and scientists have learned from scientific investigations of chronic pelvic pain syndromes (CPPS), focusing more on male pelvic pain. Many individual physicians and medical centers take a special interest in this problem and the plight of those suffering from the syndrome. The National Institutes of Health (NIH) received a directive from Congress a few years ago to pursue effective treatment modalities for CPPS and, through a consortium of national awarded medical centers, is dedicating significant efforts to new scientific studies in this endeavor. In 2008, NIH invited proposals to study in greater basic biologic detail what underlies the cause and behavior of these maladies.

CPPS exists as a nonmalignant pain emanating from structures around and inside the pelvis. There are no gold-standard objective tests that define CPPS. No one can verify and quantify the amount and intensity of pain. Only a few stalwart physicians and scientists have endeavored to uncover the possible biological basis for its existence and find any kind of rational medical treatment.

Although there are *more than two million office visits a year in the United States for complaints about prostatitis,* and although variations of this disorder make up almost 10 percent of a typical urologist's practice, such patients are sadly not the most welcomed because there are no definitive therapies to help them. Physicians want to help patients, and when they have treatments that are ineffective not only they but the patients are frustrated and dismayed. In this chapter we review the current knowledge gained from many scientific studies devoted to characterizing and managing CPPS. We also present some of the thinking that may advance our knowledge about CPPS and lead to development of new therapeutic approaches.

If one looks at the history of medicine, the pelvic malady of prostatitis was not described until the mid-nineteenth century. To our knowledge, the overwhelming number of cases diagnosed as prostatitis have never had a satisfactory remedy. Imagine all those men suffering for centuries without a clue as to what might have been going on. In the first part of the twentieth century someone introduced the theory of a possible role of bacteria and examined prostatic fluid microscopically. The secretion was cultured for the first time in 1913.

It was not until 1968, however, that Dr. Thomas Stamey and Dr. Edwin Meares at Stanford University established an appropriate, detailed patient examination that allowed the urologist to document scientifically when bacteria were truly originating from the prostate gland and not the urethra or the urinary bladder, or if there were no bacteria at all.

PROSTATITIS: A MOSTLY INCORRECT LABEL

We soon learned that bacteria were rarely the cause of CPPS, but when they were, treatment of true bacterial prostatitis was relatively easy. Chronic prostatitis is an incorrect label; we are dealing with a variable set of pain conditions with no objective markers and multivariate symptoms.

The disorder typically does not exhibit prostatocentric symptomatology, and pain sites exist between the belly button to above the midthigh. The European community has promoted the term *prostate pain syndrome* (PPS) as a more generic term over the US category label of chronic prostatitis/chronic pelvic pain syndrome (CP/CPPS). Still, they both smack of a prostatocentric approach, which is probably to be avoided for lack of evidence, and the diagnosis encourages physicians to use antibiotics as standard therapy that clearly lacks efficacy.

By definition, prostate pain syndrome is persistent discomfort or pain in the pelvic region with sterile specimen cultures and either significant or insignificant white blood cell counts in prostate specimens—semen, expressed prostatic secretion, or urine collected after prostate massage.

*In men, evidence of inflammation in the prostate
by itself and with no infection present offers
little help in guiding any effective therapy for
symptoms of pelvic pain and dysfunction in men.*

There does not appear to be any diagnostic or therapeutic advantage to differentiating between those patients with significant or insignificant white blood cells from the prostate. Remarkably, in the authors' experience, men with *no prostate inflammation* appear to suffer more and longer-lasting pelvic pain on average. *We believe that chronic testicular pain should be included in the general term of chronic pelvic pain syndrome or CPPS.* Women with pelvic pain, particularly interstitial cystitis-type pain, fall under a general diagnostic designation termed bladder pain syndrome (BPS). In this chapter we use prostate pain syndrome or CPPS as a model to discuss scientific investigations and treatments.

DISCOVERING THE CULPRIT IN PELVIC PAIN

Our viewpoint about prostatitis/CPPS differs from the conventional practice of routinely identifying and treating pelvic pain in men as a prostate infection. *We do not see the prostate as the source of the problem of most male pelvic pain.* What we have proposed for many years has to do with our view of the anatomical areas of the pelvis that actually cause the pain and how that pain is created.

Of course, all pain messages transmit through *sensory nerve receptors, then coalesce into fine webs of nerves ending in the spinal cord and, ultimately, forwarded to the brain,* where they are perceived and interpreted in different ways by each patient. Physicians traditionally assign *blame for pain to the various organs of the pelvis*—the uterus, the vagina, the testicles, the penis, the prostate gland, and excretory organs such as the rectum and urinary bladder—rather than suspecting the supportive structures of these organs—connective tissue such as ligaments and tendons, muscles, blood vessels, and nerves serving these structures.

There is also the phenomenon known as "referral," whereby pain coming from an organ may not be felt in the organ itself but can be felt in remote areas, including the skin. Because of the intimate relationship between the nerves, a strong signal from one area may stimulate a neighboring nerve, even though that neighbor nerve was not being irritated by the stimulus. This represents the method by which muscles become tense even though they are not related to the source of irritation.

> *There are twenty-plus different muscles*
> *and a widespread distribution of*
> *nerves in and around the pelvis.*

These muscles and nerves obviously play an indispensable role in association with the organs they support.

UNDERSTANDING THE MUSCLES
OF THE PELVIC FLOOR

As the myriad nerves interlace throughout the pelvis, the stimulating nerves responsible for smooth muscle contraction and organ function, as well as the motor nerves that control supporting muscles, balance and complement each other. We divide muscles into smooth muscle and striated muscle. Smooth muscles exist in the walls of the intestines and provide the motility of our intestinal function; similarly, the urinary bladder, the uterus, the ejaculatory ducts, the prostate, and even the heart function with various types of smooth muscle. Our skeletal or striated muscles are responsible for voluntary movements and offer support and balance to the pelvic structures.

It can be difficult to understand the dull and diffuse nature of pelvic pain unless you understand how nerves work and realize that there can be communication between nerves (cross-talk) as well as intermingling of signals from various nerves that can confuse someone about where the pain really originates.

Adrenaline, in the form of a biochemical called norepinephrine, stimulates smooth muscle through the adrenaline receptors embedded in the muscles. These receptors *are extremely sensitive to small amounts of norepinephrine*. We designate these smooth muscle receptors as alpha and beta receptors. The heart is full of beta receptors, for example, and when one is excited, even mentally, adrenaline causes the heart to go into a racing configuration. *The smooth muscles in the pelvis,* while confined primarily to the organs, *respond in the same way to mental signals that release adrenaline* and cause a reaction in the pelvic muscles. *There are also adrenaline receptors in the contracting or striated muscles* of the pelvis that can be excited by release of excitatory biochemical substances like adrenaline—these are responsible for the "fight or flight" response that gives us extra energy. This is why people can sometimes perform heroic maneuvers in stressful situations.

Dr. Steven Kaplan and colleagues at Columbia University reported that the inappropriate contraction of the external urinary sphincter during voiding can be misdiagnosed as chronic prostatitis. An interesting observation in their review was that 91 percent of the subjects in this study were firstborn sons. Dr. Kaplan's group felt that behavioral modification and biofeedback to teach the appropriate relaxation approach to urinating were good therapeutic options.

SYMPTOMS OF CHRONIC PROSTATITIS

Chronic prostatitis means different things to patients and doctors. It is a common diagnosis—one of the most common genitourinary diagnoses of men under fifty years—*though clearly a misnomer. The primary symptomatic complaint that becomes chronic is pelvic pain or discomfort.* Patients may or may not have accompanying urinary and sexual problems as well.

Frequently the pain during urination or during or after ejaculation is associated with the urinary or sexual problems. The physician and patient need to understand the circumstances at the time of onset, how long-occurring and cyclic the discomfort has been, what degree of intensity is involved, and where the pain is located. We also evaluate the patient's attitude toward his pain, whether the pain is variable or constant, and if he is having pain-free intervals.

> *Three cardinal symptoms are associated*
> *with the diagnosis of chronic prostatitis—*
> *pelvic pain and discomfort, disturbances in*
> *urination, and disturbed sexual function.*

The second set of common symptoms are *disturbances of urination—* typically lower urinary tract symptoms such as a sense of urinary urgency and frequency, inhibition of the ability to release the urine, a burning sensation, or dysuria, with voiding, and depressed flow. There may be dribbling of urine at the end of emptying the bladder because of poor balance between the sphincter muscles and the contraction of the bladder, often resulting in "trapping" of urine within the urethra as it runs through the prostate.

> *In men, sometimes there is a spasm-like*
> *discomfort immediately after ejaculation*
> *or a discomfort that lasts as a nagging or*
> *aching sensation for several hours or days.*

The third set of symptoms is *disturbances in sexual function* that may include loss of libido or sex drive, inability to attain or maintain erection for satisfying sexual intercourse, and, most important, discomfort with ejaculation. There may be changes in the spermatic fluid such as decrease in volume, blood staining on occasion, and watery or clumpy, discolored semen.

MEDICAL HISTORY

The typical patient is a young to middle-aged man with variable symptoms of chronic, irritative, and obstructive voiding accompanied by moderate to severe pain in the pelvis, low back, perineum, and genitalia. To qualify as chronic pelvic pain, the condition should occur longer than six months and, for research purposes, be continuous within the previous three months.

The patient is understandably tense, wary, and defensive, having encountered frustration and rejection previously. The physician should listen to the patient's complaints and accurately document the circumstances surrounding the onset of the disorder—sensory descriptions, various treatment modalities, and outcomes, noting particularly the time course of events and associated triggers that may have caused a flare in his symptoms. The US national cohort study by the NIH reported a typical duration of patient complaints averaging four years.

The urologist's first order of business when referred a man diagnosed with prostatitis/chronic pelvic pain syndrome is to accept the challenge seriously and treat the man suffering with this condition with respect, interest, and compassion.

The urologist evaluating pelvic pain in a male must rule out associated urinary bladder or prostate diseases. Errors in diagnosis and inappropriate therapeutic pathways may ensue if a less-than-systematic evaluation is undertaken. Both prostate and bladder cancer as well as urinary stone disease have been missed because of an inappropriate diagnosis of "chronic prostatitis." It is crucial to have empathy for the suffering patient, documenting his description of the physical characteristics of the pain complex: What makes it worse, what helps, where is the pain referred, and what associations exist with sexual function? The psychosexual behavior and influence of sexual partner relationships play a significant role. How has the chronic pain affected libido, the ability to attain adequate penile erections, accomplish intercourse, reach orgasm, and have pleasurable ejaculation?

Associated alimentary tract complaints such as irritable bowel disorder, constipation, dietary exacerbations, and bowel function may point to further clarifying aspects of the disorder. Further, the psychosocial medical history should probe for genetic or acquired personality types: tense, anxious, chronic tension-holding patterns, possible childhood issues of sexual or physical abuse, traumatic toilet training, abnormal bowel patterns, teen sexual problems, excessive masturbation, suppressed homosexuality, excessive weight lifting, gymnastic maneuvers, and activities such as dance training.

In our research we utilize symptom questionnaires and validated instruments to detail patient psychological issues. These tools help quantify the baseline, eventual progress, and outcome of our management techniques. The most widely used research tool is the National Institutes of Health Chronic Prostatitis Symptom Index (NIH-CPSI). This widely used symptom scoring analyzes pain, urinary symptoms, and quality of life as three separate domains. Almost every meaningful clinical trial of treatment has used this scoring system to evaluate efficacy outcome. We state the percent improvement in the CPSI score when available in the treatment studies described below. The CPSI has also been modified by Dr. Clemens from Michigan to allow symptom scoring for women. An alternate type of CPPS symptom questionnaire—the Stanford Pelvic Pain Symptom Score (PPSS)—has also been useful to us, although it is not usually reported in scientific studies. The PPSS expands the description of named painful anatomical locations and grades the severity of pain at each site (0 to 4+); it includes urinary symptoms that mimic the International Prostate Symptom Score (IPSS) and scores sexual dysfunction aspects of the patient's condition as a separate domain. Our group utilizes both symptom-scoring questionnaires in the treatment outcome analysis of CPPS therapy.

THE PHYSICIAN'S EXAMINATION

When physicians examine a patient *they typically focus on the organs* of the pelvis; they perform a rectal or vaginal examination and attempt to palpate the uterus, the ovaries, the rectum, the prostate, the bladder, and testicles, but they usually *ignore the important integration of the muscles and the fascia or ligaments holding these organs.*

It is our duty to elicit with the examination what the patient experiences and to attempt to correlate what we find with any possible abnormality that may be occurring either in the organs or in the pelvic muscles. This is not a simple task. The majority of patients suffering with chronic pelvic pain have no classic standard findings that can be easily detected. However, certain basic urologic evaluations should be done, including a careful lower-body neurologic examination, urinalysis, and a serum prostate-specific antigen (PSA) test in men over fifty.

*It is our considered view that in evaluating
a patient with chronic pelvic pain it is
imperative to do a thorough evaluation of the
muscles and ligaments of the pelvic floor.*

In our evaluation at Stanford, like most urologists, we examine the prostate for microorganisms and inflammatory white blood cells. This requires the patient to urinate a small amount prior to examination so that we can compare this sample microscopically to what may be found in voided urine after massage of the prostate. We palpate the pelvic muscles, looking for actual trigger points or specific discomfort zones, especially surrounding the prostate. We then feel the prostate gland itself; we determine its consistency, whether it is soft or "boggy," and whether there are areas of induration or hardness—which may represent fibrosis or scarring from previous inflammation—but we must remain ever vigilant for cancer.

We methodically massage the prostate gland, beginning at the base and milking it toward the center on each side to express prostatic fluid into the urethra. The prostate gland is composed of twenty to thirty small microscopic tunnels (acini) emanating from the periphery of the prostate. Each glandular unit is connected to the outside world by a pinpoint duct that opens into the urethra on each side of the main seminal vesicles' ejaculatory duct located in the center of the prostate. These tiny ducts expel the enzyme-rich prostatic secretion with smooth muscle prostate contractions at the time of sexual ejaculation.

The easiest way to perform this pelvic examination is with the patient lying supine with the legs spread in stirrups (the female position). This allows the examiner to have leverage and direct visualization of the penis and the urethral opening to collect prostatic fluid. We have found it convenient to collect the fluid with a tiny sterile glass pipette, the prostatic secretion drops accumulating with capillary action as they appear at the penis opening or meatus, particularly when there are only one or two drops that are quite precious to be able to examine and culture.

Once the prostatic fluid has been collected, the patient will urinate a small volume to provide a washout of prostatic fluid that can be separated, analyzed, and submitted for bacterial culture. This is particularly important when no prostatic fluid is expressed. We advise patients to refrain from any sexual ejaculation for seven days prior to coming in for the examination to afford a better opportunity to maximize collection of prostatic fluid. Older men typically have more prostatic fluid because the gland is larger. Younger men find it a challenge to refrain from sex for a week.

Unfortunately, careful analysis of the prostatic fluid is usually performed only in academic or university medical centers where an intellectual curiosity prevails.

We take the patient's prostatic fluid to our office laboratory, where a simple examination under the microscope (after staining the fluid with a dye) helps identify white cells and improves the analysis. We count the number of white cells in the prostatic fluid to compare with counts from normal, asymptomatic men and to track changes as a treatment program is instituted.

HOW COMMON IS INFECTIOUS PROSTATITIS?

Acute bacterial prostatitis, as described earlier, is a fairly easy diagnosis to make. It is associated with pain in the prostate, difficulty urinating, high fever, chills, and weakness. It is serious because bacteria can spread into the bloodstream, causing sepsis or blood poisoning. Acute bacterial prostatitis requires aggressive antimicrobial therapy and sometimes needs catheter drainage of the urinary tract. Inadequately treated acute bacterial prostatitis may potentially become dormant and develop into *recurrent* chronic bacterial prostatitis. We typically treat acute prostatitis for a total of twenty-eight days using potent antibiotics. We administer antibiotics for about six weeks when true chronic bacterial infection is established through a microbiology laboratory.

> *Chronic prostatitis is caused by bacteria in*
> *only 5 percent of cases of pelvic pain.*

There has been much debate about whether chronic pelvic pain represents an infectious disease. The consensus of expert opinion today is that chronic prostatitis, as a medical disorder, is probably caused directly by microbial agents in only about 5 percent of the cases. Most of these episodes of bacterial prostatitis are without symptoms between infection flare-ups. Men who complain of chronic pelvic pain and who have been diagnosed with prostatitis may possess increased bacterial counts found in the prostatic fluid. But the bacteria are normal flora, or normal types of bacteria in the urethra, and they colonize the prostate ducts in low numbers, just as we find normal resident bacteria in the vagina, the mouth, the rectum, and other parts of the body. Uropathogens, however, are bacteria not normally found in the genitourinary (GU) tract and are known to be invasive and to cause inflammation of both the prostate and bladder. These bacteria are organisms from the intestinal tract. When a physician identifies significant numbers of these bacteria in the genitourinary system, in the urethra, the bladder, or coming from the prostate gland itself, he or she considers this to be bacterial cause of the symptoms. Are we not trying hard enough to find poorly detected microorganisms that may be responsible for inciting this condition? Some have suggested we should culture the body fluids for a longer time to detect the slow-growing bacteria that may also be hiding out under biofilms. Dr. Ronald Cohen, a pathologist from Australia, has just produced evidence that acne organisms can be found in the prostate if carefully cultured. The presence of the bacteria was sleuthed out using DNA tracking. It appears that those individuals who suffer from CPPS do indeed have a higher incidence of the positive DNA fingerprints when you take biopsies from their prostates compared with men who never had CPPS, but as we discuss below, this appears to be irrelevant to their symptoms.

Serious investigators have looked at multiple microorganisms that might be the cause of chronic prostatitis, including microbial forms such as *Chlamydia, Ureaplasma,* and even parasites or protozoans such as *Trichomonas.* Dr. Andrew Doble and associates from England performed an exhaustive search for infectious agents in chronic prostatitis syndromes using ultrasound-guided tissue biopsies of the prostate. They found that 88 percent of their patients had chronic inflammation in the tissue, but only 15 percent of patients had any organisms that were cultured or grew from the tissue, and actually these were considered to be contaminants from the skin. This information again reinforces the concept that we are dealing with a painful disorder and no proven microorganism as a cause. Unfortunately, most physicians and patients believe chronic prostatitis to be an infectious entity and are searching for the Holy Grail of antimicrobial treatment that will once and for all eradicate these pesky organisms from the patient's system. We believe this is a fruitless quest.

*While very small percentages (3–10 percent)
of patients have been found to carry certain
unusual organisms, there have never been
convincing studies to prove that these organisms
are specific causative agents in prostatitis.*

Another controversy that continues to be debated among urologists and microbiologists is whether *gram-positive organisms* (a laboratory stain classification) such as *Staphylococcus* and beta strep, commonly found as normal flora in the urethra, may indeed act as pathogenic bacteria or organisms that would invade and cause inflammation. These gram-positive microbes are usually found on the skin and in the mouth, as opposed to gram-negative microbes that come from the large intestine. While some patients may have large numbers of these organisms in the urethra and colonizing the prostate, use of antimicrobials to eradicate the organisms does not seem to provide improvement in symptoms, and there is very little association with the cause and effect of symptoms.

Dr. Wolfgang Weidner from the University of Giessen in Germany is an important contributor to evaluating the occurrence of microorganisms and inflammation in CPPS. He published a paper in 1991 demonstrating a thorough search for microorganisms in hundreds of consecutive patients. He found high numbers of bacteria and several sub-bacterial species of *Ureaplasma* in a typical prostatitis pattern associated with increased numbers of white cells in the prostatic secretion. At that time he felt there was an important difference in the classification between patients with and without inflammation in the prostatic fluid and that there were differences in the symptoms from those patients that had no white cells and pain in the prostate (the NIH classification difference between IIIA and IIIB).

Our own anecdotal experience suggests a difference between the two categories in symptoms and in response to therapy. However, *a careful NIH-sponsored study concluded that there was no correlation between evidence of infection or inflammation in the prostate and the symptoms of pros-*

tatitis/chronic pelvic pain. The precise relationship of prostate inflammation and chronic pelvic pain remains to be elucidated.

THE INFLAMMATION DEBATE

In the first place, we have only small shreds of evidence that inflammation may be involved in causing the pain of CPPS. Even less well understood is what biologic or physical entity may be inciting the inflammation. In a few instances, some tissue has been available for sampling—bladder, prostate, rectum, vagina—and no obvious microbiologic substance appears to be an initiator. Furthermore, the presence and degree of inflammation do not correlate quantitatively with the degree of pain.

The occurrence of infection/inflammation in chronic prostatitis/CPPS fails to be consistent and is not helpful in diagnostic terms. Dr. John McNeal, a research pathologist at Stanford University, worked on prostate disease, particularly prostate cancer, his whole professional life; he found many years ago that *between 5 and 15 percent of men over the age of sixty have inflammation in their prostate tissue on microscopic examination but absolutely no complaint of pelvic pain.* An NIH study found no relationship between infection/inflammation and severity of pain and dysfunction in prostatitis.

Doctors can determine that there is inflammation in the prostate ducts when they look at expressed prostatic secretion under the microscope at four hundred times magnification. However, it is not always possible to massage prostatic fluid from a patient. We then must rely on a postmassage voided urine specimen and separate prostatic fluid by centrifugation from the urine for analysis. Again, our male patients with prostatitis who have high numbers of inflammatory white cells in their expressed prostatic secretion actually seem to have less pain on average than those with few or no white blood cells coming from the ducts of the prostate. There is no current scientific information to explain why this is so.

As we do not have proof of infectious agents causing chronic pelvic pain syndrome, the unanswered question remains: What is causing the inflammation? Many investigators believe that it has to do with *dysfunction of the voiding mechanism*: an imbalance in the urinary muscle control causes reflux or pressure of urine and hence toxic substances of urine backing up into the prostate gland ducts to create an inflammatory and irritated condition. In simple language, tension in the pelvic muscles may be inhibiting the free flow of urine, causing it to reflux or back up into the prostate.

Dr. Linda Shortliffe, a urologist at Stanford, performed an analysis of the prostatic fluid proteins in an attempt to look at differences between men with bacterial and nonbacterial prostatitis. She reported that even patients without bacterial prostatitis could have elevated levels of prostatic immunoglobulins, the body's response to infection or inflammation. In 1995, Dr. Robert Nadler reported the effect of inflammation on prostate-specific antibody (PSA) levels—the enzyme blood test used to test for the possible presence of prostate cancer. The presence of inflammation was quite common, and nearly all of the men with high PSA levels had at least one biopsy specimen positive for chronic inflammation. Confusing the issue, however, 77 percent of those with normal PSA levels also had small areas of inflammation on biopsy. In many cases, acute and chronic inflammation were more prevalent in the high-PSA group (63 percent, versus 27 percent in the normal PSA group). Nadler concluded that a quantitative demonstration of acute and chronic inflammation in the tissue was not necessarily associated with clinical bacterial prostatitis, or even symptoms, but might be an important contributor to elevated PSA levels in the blood.

Immune response may occur with nerve growth factors and associated inflammatory agents known as cytokines, and this raises some intriguing possibilities. First, it may reveal biological markers that could be analyzed to show an abnormal presence and provide potential therapeutic blocking agents for the inflammatory condition. Very small amounts of nerve growth factor, perhaps released because of primary prostate nerve damage, can increase sensitivity to both thermal and mechanical stimulation. These chemical changes relate to altered sensitivity to pain and could be responsible for the dynamics of fluctuation in this chronic pain syndrome. Not finding an elusive inflammatory inciting agent or evidence of obvious inflammation does not detract from our belief and supporting evidence that the central nervous system—the brain and spinal cord—in conjunction with powerful immune-regulating mechanisms known as the hypothalamus-pituitary-adrenal (HPA) axis may be intimately involved in altering inflammatory events in the body related to CPPS. Neurogenic inflammation (inflammation resulting from the local release of biochemical substances from nerves) is a phenomenon that has been demonstrated in many experimental models. It is clear that the autonomic nervous system, particularly the adrenergic or sympathetic system, plays a very important role. Sensory nerve endings are activated and then release cytokines and many other inflammatory mediators, which in turn affect the surrounding tissue.

Small microvessels dilate and become permeable, blood flow increases (causing redness), and exuding blood plasma allows white blood cells to accumulate. This is acute inflammation. This inflammatory process may, in turn, excite or activate the stress system, causing anxiety and recycling the neurogenic inflammation. The hallmark of chronic inflammation is infiltration of tissue with mononuclear inflammatory cells ("mononuclear cells," "round cells," i.e., monocytes, lymphocytes, and/or plasma cells). Generally, good tissue has been (and is being) destroyed, and there will be some evidence of healing (scarring, fibroblast proliferation, new blood vessel proliferation).

We label the fields that explore these relationships and pathophysiological phenomena *psychoneuroimmunology* and *psychoneuroendocrinology*. This book cannot serve as the forum to expound on the multiple scientific studies on these issues. We must, however, always hold our beliefs in abeyance and remain open-minded about the possibilities in our quest to understand this CPPS malady.

IMAGING OF THE PROSTATE IN CHRONIC PROSTATITIS

The best way to look at the prostate gland tissue is to use *transrectal ultrasound* (TRUS). This method of evaluation can often be quite valuable in demonstrating inflamed tissue, the presence of stones in the ducts (representing urinary mineral deposits), swelling and thickening of seminal vesicles (semen storage organs behind the prostate), and accurate measurement of the size of the gland. Japanese investigators have used computerized x-ray images and angiography or dye in blood vessels to evaluate chronic pelvic pain. They demonstrated excellent three-dimensional graphic images of veins around the prostate and found considerable congestion in these veins behind the bladder and along the sides of the prostate in patients suffering with pain. In these patients, the veins on the surface of the prostate were much thicker in diameter than those in subjects with no pain. This basically represents varicose veins of the prostate. It is suggestive of heightened tension in the muscles of the pelvic floor and is supportive of our view that chronic pelvic pain syndromes are associated with muscle tension.

> *There is rarely, if ever, any obvious inflammation on the surface of the prostatic urethra in the condition of prostatitis.*

It is quite common for urologists to look inside the urethra, prostate, and bladder in patients suffering from this disorder with a technique called *cystoscopy*. This consists of passing a pencil-sized flexible probe with magnifying optical lenses, high-intensity fiber-optic light, and associated video camera up the penile urethra. However, cystoscopy may be the least productive procedure that can be done. Some urologists will say to the patient, "Oh, yes, I see some inflammation in the prostate." This is anatomically impossible, because they are looking only at the surface of the urethra and not at the prostatic tissue itself.

We should mention the theory that the compression, stretching, or entrapment of pudendal nerves in the pelvis is a potential cause of chronic pelvic pain. Some propose five essential criteria for such a diagnosis: (1) pain along the anatomical distribution of the pudendal nerve; (2) the pain aggravated by sitting; (3) the patient is not awakened at night by the pain; (4) there is no objective sensory loss on clinical examination; and (5) the pain is improved by an anesthetic pudendal nerve block. Neurophysiologic tests such as pudendal nerve motor latency test and EMG may serve as complementary diagnostic measures.

*Controversial surgical procedures
for pelvic pain have produced little
convincing evidence as to efficacy.*

Patients thought to have this syndrome typically have considerable pain while sitting that is then completely relieved when standing. It is also relieved by sitting on a toilet seat, although both of these criteria exist to some degree in pelvic pain syndrome. There are theories that athletic endeavors may have caused distortion in the nerve pathway. Similarly, chronic constipation may contribute to the presumed condition.

We do not recommend pudendal nerve injections or pudendal nerve surgery. Certainly, any surgical approach to alleviate this condition must rely on documentation of nerve dysfunction as measured by nerve conduction studies. It appears, however, that less than 50 percent of patients experience any reduction of their pain with surgery.

*In our experience, most patients undergoing
surgical procedures for muscle-based pelvic pain
regret such procedures and often report less-
than-satisfactory results, a high level of new
symptoms, and compromised pelvic floor stability.*

We have never seen a patient whose symptoms have resolved after pudendal nerve entrapment surgery.

ISOLATED MALE ORCHIALGIA
(PAIN IN THE TESTICLES)

Chronic orchialgia, or pain in the testes, vexes a lot of young men, and they reluctantly bring this to the attention of their physician. Testicular pain occurs most commonly in men in their twenties and thirties and requires careful history and physical examination because this is also the age group where testicular cancer most commonly occurs. Usually the examination is negative, with a complaint of pain localization to one side or the other, and when the head of the epididymis organ is squeezed it reproduces the pain for the patient. Rarely does a vasectomy result in such tenderness or chronic orchialgia. It is important to understand the nerve supply to the testes so that the diagnostic evaluation can make some functional sense. The pelvic nerve plexus supplies the input, and pain can arise from both the normal sensory nerves and the autonomic nerves. These fibers are carried in the branches of the genitofemoral and ilioinguinal nerves. Findings of fluid around the testicle, varicose veins, or sperm cysts (spermatoceles) are usually coincidental and are never the cause of the chronic orchialgia. This pain is almost always spermatic cord/epididymal nerve pain and not testicular pain.

*Removal of the epididymis for treating
chronic testes pain has met with failure.*

Slightly more successful when all else has failed has been cutting the nerves, using a microscopic method, to remove all nerve fibers from the spermatic cord arising from the testicular tissue or the scrotal contents. We always perform a selective anesthetic spermatic cord nerve block as a diagnostic and sometimes therapeutic procedure first, adding a cortisone solution to a long-acting anesthetic. Several of these nerve blocks at intervals can sometimes relieve the cyclical nature of this syndrome. A recent report by Dr. Magdy Hassouna from Canada proposes that sacral nerve root electrical stimulation may be beneficial in these patients, and in some cases skin surface electrical stimulation has been helpful.

URODYNAMICS

One investigative tool to evaluate urinary and prostate function consists of physiological measurements with a procedure called *urodynamics*. Such testing should be suggested only if it would benefit the physician to understand and treat specific abnormalities. This testing procedure evaluates physiologic function of smooth and striated muscle function in the bladder, prostate, and urinary sphincters. We place a small pressure-sensing catheter in the bladder to detect changes in bladder pressure; the catheter simultaneously monitors the urethral voluntary sphincter pressure activity and associated pelvic floor function. An important component of this testing includes a catheter balloon in the rectum to monitor abdominal pressure. We utilize electrical sensors patched to the skin around the anal muscles to detect electrical activity within the pelvic floor, both with relaxation and voluntary contraction, but primarily to determine how much relaxation is achieved when the patient is attempting to urinate. For decades studies have compared symptoms and morphological, microbiological, and urodynamic findings in patients with CPPS. A common theme emerges suggesting *functional* obstruction at the level of the bladder neck and external sphincter, high sensitivity during filling, and poor or interrupted urinary flow. Abnormally low urinary flow rates are found in 65 percent of patients. Some patients respond to alpha-nerve blocking agents as therapy for CPPS, but most do not.

MUSCLE TENSION AND CHRONIC PELVIC PAIN SYNDROME

Because we have so little to document a cause of chronic pelvic pain, theories and partial bits of evidence are discussed interminably.

Clearly, we need evidence for specific treatment, but multimodal shotgun therapy still prevails. Many investigators publish articles reviewing the evidence for abnormalities and potential treatment approaches, but progress requires strong scientific studies. Fortunately the NIH, through its National Institute of Diabetes and Digestive and Kidney Diseases, is providing funding for cooperative basic science and translational investigation, and we hope this gathering of the minds will bear fruit.

A study published in 1987 by Dr. Wayne Hellstrom and colleagues from the University of California, San Francisco, promoted this concept with case reports. Their physiologic studies revealed elevated urethral pressures where the urinary channel runs through the middle of the prostate, causing reflux of urine minerals and toxic metabolites into the peripheral or outer zone of the prostate, the location of most of the inflammation. The peripheral zone ducts are perpendicular to the course of the urethra and are susceptible to high pressure in the prostate. Specific measurements of intraprostatic pressure have been undertaken in patients suffering from chronic prostate pain, and one series of forty-two patients showed significant elevation of prostate hydrostatic pressures.

> *With regard to inflammation of the prostate,*
> *it is our view that tension myalgia and*
> *chronic pelvic pain syndromes leading to*
> *imbalance in urinary function can cause mild*
> *inflammation in the prostate. For this reason*
> *treating inflammation is of little help because*
> *inflammation is an effect and not a cause.*

Dr. George Barbalias from Greece proposes this mechanistic cause of chronic prostatitis. He advocated long ago the use of potent alpha-receptor blockade as a method of treatment. He actually used needle electrodes to measure electrical signals from the external urethral sphincter. While he found normal motor unit potentials in the majority of the patients and discovered that there was a coordinated function of the bladder and the external sphincter during voiding with no difference between inflammatory and noninflammatory patients, both groups had decreased urinary flow rate. He said this was a *functional* urethral obstruction but not an actual physical obstruction. This *functional* urethral obstruction represents chronic pelvic muscle tension.

Dr. Dirk-Henrik Zermann and colleagues at the University of Colorado in Denver showed that in men with chronic pelvic pain there was a strong association with neuromuscular and myofascial (muscles and ligaments) dysfunction. In a clinical evaluation of 103 patients seen at their clinic, 91 men (88.3 percent) had abnormal tenderness of the striated or voluntary muscle of the pelvis, and this myofascial tenderness was virtually always associated with inability to relax the pelvic floor efficiently. Diane Hetrick, a physiotherapist, and the team with Dr. Richard Berger at the University of Washington in Seattle have confirmed the opinion that musculoskeletal dysfunction occurs in men with chronic pelvic pain syndrome.

A higher likelihood of increased pelvic floor muscle tone, pain with internal palpation, and increased tension and pain with external palpation was found in patients with CPPS as compared with healthy controls.

Furthermore, these investigators at Washington showed hypersensitivity in the pelvic (perineal area) sensory nerves of patients. They used a flash heat technique to create a painful heat stimulus in the perineum. When compared with healthy volunteers, patients suffering from chronic pelvic pain syndrome definitely showed more sensitivity to the heat pain.

Many physician specialists (rheumatologists/immunologists) working with arthritis believe that the primary abnormality leading to expression of symptoms in fibromyalgia and related conditions consists of errant central nervous system function. This concept promotes the idea that there may be skeletal muscle abnormalities in patients having pain.

CENTRAL NERVOUS SYSTEM STRESS AND CPPS

Throughout the years, many physicians have noted the contributions of stress or anxiety to pelvic pain syndromes. In 1986 a group from Sweden (led by Lars Gatenbeck) studied rats that were stimulated and stressed with or without hormone additives. They investigated the microscopic changes of the prostate under these conditions. Inflammation of the gland was thought to occur because of stress reactions increasing output of adrenaline and other biochemical neurotransmitters.

In their experiments, rats were submitted to stress stimuli for ten days. Examination of the prostate tissue after this kind of activity demonstrated moderate infiltration of inflammatory cells—there was a significant difference between rats that received stimulation and rats that did not, with the latter having little or no inflammation. At the same time, they found a reduced serum testosterone level, but it was not clear what the influence or importance of this hormonal change could be. The other feature noted was that the lobes of the rat prostate having the least advanced drainage system had a greater involvement in inflammatory manifestation. This is an example of one of the very few experimental attempts to document the behavioral effects on both physiologic and microscopic changes.

Dr. Miller's psychological approach alone
improved the condition of 86 percent
of his patients with prostatitis.

In 1988 Dr. Harry C. Miller studied 218 men who had complaints typical of CPPS. Sixty percent or 134 of these patients were followed carefully and managed only with stress control. With this psychological approach alone, 86 percent of the patients reported that they were better, much better, or cured. Most important, repeat cultures, prostatic massages, instrumentation, and medications were not utilized at all in this group of patients, as Miller relied solely on stress management.

CORTISOL AND CPPS

We recently studied a group of forty-five men with CPPS and twenty normal age-matched men and found the patients to have significantly more perceived stress and anxiety. These men were also found to produce a more rapid rise in morning awakening levels of cortisol in their saliva. We then followed up on this phenomenon and invited these patients to come in for acute stress testing in the laboratory. Compared with the normal control men, our patients showed a *depressed* afternoon ability of the brain to produce the precursor (ACTH) for cortisol production from the adrenal glands compared with normal control men. Perhaps the blunting of cortisol of men with CPPS in the afternoon represents the fatigue of the cortisol production machinery of the brain.

TREATMENTS AND CLINICAL TRIALS

The NIH promotes clinical research regarding the pervasive disorder of chronic prostatitis and chronic pelvic pain syndrome. They want to find a satisfactory treatment. Progress in treatment requires documentation of results with strong levels of evidence that something works. The best level of evidence occurs when patients are treated with an active drug or treatment method and a similar group is randomized to be treated with a sham procedure or placebo drug and not to know it. We call this a blinded control clinical research trial. These are very expensive and difficult to perform. Sometimes it is impossible to blind patients from knowing that they are not receiving the real thing.

PHARMACEUTICALS

A good example in a recent nationwide study evaluated the two most common medication treatments for the disorder: oral ciprofloxacin

(Cipro), a potent fluoroquinolone antibiotic, and/or oral tamsulosin (Flomax), a potent alpha–nerve receptor blocking agent for the smooth muscle of the prostate and urethra. These two pharmacologic agents were tested in a blinded fashion against a placebo or sugar pill as a treatment of these syndromes. This was an important study because no one had ever systematically evaluated the effect of antibiotics for these "nonbacterial" disorders, although many doctors and patients claimed improvement.

Cipro, Flomax, Lyrica, and Uroxatral are
no better than placebo for CPPS.

The outcome of the study showed that the symptom scores improved slightly regardless of whether the patients took the antibiotic, the alpha blocker, or the placebo. The contribution of an alpha-blocking smooth muscle relaxant continues to be debated with regard to its efficacy. In our own practice, virtually every patient who comes to see us has been previously treated with potent antibiotics or alpha blocking agents, or both, but they continue to have recurrent complaints. Further testing patients with shorter-term CPPS with an additional randomized clinical trial of another alpha blocker, alfuzosin (Uroxatral), demonstrated no difference over a placebo. Finally, a recent study of pregabalin (Lyrica) as an oral treatment for CPPS was not found to be any better than a sugar placebo when taken over several weeks.

Oral medications for pelvic pain continue
to produce disappointing results.

Dr. Daniel Shoskes investigated the use of an herbal dietary supplement known as a bioflavonoid. Quercetin was given to patients with chronic prostatitis/CPPS in a blinded fashion for one month. Patients taking the substance had their symptom scores decrease from 21 to 13 (67 percent improvement). This therapy seems to be well tolerated and offers significant symptomatic improvement in many men with chronic pelvic pain syndrome. Larger national studies need to be performed for a high level of scientific evidence. Another herbal approach from Europe suggests that a formulation of rye grass pollen (Cernilton) has some anti-inflammatory effects and has been popular as treatment for nonbacterial prostatitis. A well-done study from Germany evaluated the primary outcome of treatment (change in pelvic pain) over a twelve-week period. In a group of 139 patients, half on pollen and half on placebo, the pollen group dropped their pain scores an average of 45 percent and the placebo group an average of 29 percent.

What about acupuncture and electrical stimulation therapy? Drs. R. C. Chen and J. C. Nickel reported in 2003 that acupuncture treatments given twice weekly for six weeks improved total CPSI and pain scores by 70 percent on average. This was a small study in twelve men with no placebo control. A more recent trial was reported from Turkey in 2010. Ninety-seven patients received six weekly acupuncture treatments, and at twenty-four weeks follow-up the total CPSI score improved by 57 percent and the pelvic pain score by 45 percent. Another percutaneous needle study, also from Turkey, tested the efficiency of posterior tibial nerve (at the ankle) stimulation in CPPS. They had eighty-nine patients randomized to needle electrical stimulation or sham thirty minutes once weekly for twelve weeks. Success was defined as a 50 percent decrease in pain scores, and 66 percent of the patients achieved this level of relief at the end of twelve weeks. Of course, electrical stimulation therapy like this cannot be done easily on a long-term basis. The same holds true for internal pelvic high-frequency local electrical stimulation, which was tried on eighty-eight patients in Switzerland. Electrode catheters were placed into the prostatic urethra as well as the anal canal. Stimulation was performed for thirty minutes twice weekly for five weeks. The CPSI total score and pain improved 52 percent by the end of therapy, but symptoms recurred by three months later.

Obviously the most convenient way to apply electrical stimulation would be surface or transcutaneous electrical nerve stimulation (TENS). When twenty-four patients were treated with this technique, with electrode pads applied to the pubic and perineal area and treatment given for twenty minutes daily, five times a week for four weeks, the CPSI scores improved 45 percent. Patients receiving antibiotics improved their scores by 22 percent. This trial requires sham treatments and longer follow-up.

What about electrical stimulation using permanently implanted electrodes? Dr. Steven Siegel from Minnesota implanted small electrodes (Medtronic InterStim) through the posterior skin and sacral bone openings to stimulate the sacral nerves in nine women and one man. He documented an average 53 percent decrease in pain on a simple pain scale, but there were twenty-seven minor complications associated with the implantation procedure.

Heat therapy (hyperthermia) is not an approach we advocate. Some studies have reported favorable results. Thermal therapy consists of various forms of heat induction—microwave, radio frequency, laser, and ultrasound energy—where, in place of "cutting" tissue as in surgery, the prostate tissue is heated to a temperature that may cause tissue destruction. A publication in 1993 described fifty-four patients who had significant prostatitis symptoms for a period of over two years despite several courses of antimicrobial or anti-inflammatory therapy with no significant clinical benefit. The method of treatment utilized transrectal hyperthermia, and the target temperature was only 42.5°C, therefore not creating any significant damage of tissue. Transrectal ultrasound could not detect changes in the prostate volume or shape after the procedure. Overall, 50 percent of the patients reported an improvement in the quality of life; 47 percent reported no change. *This would be consistent with a strong placebo effect.* In 1994 Dr. J. C. Nickel reported using transurethral microwave thermal therapy at higher temperatures ranging from 45 to 60°C that do cause death of prostatic tissue. Patients with nonbacterial prostatitis showed significant reductions in their symptom severity indices; 47 percent had a marked improvement at three months. A similar study utilized cooled transurethral thermal therapy on thirty-five men in 2004 in the United Kingdom. These investigators found 51 percent improvement in the CPSI total score and 60 percent improvement at twelve months of follow-up. However, this *again is not far from what one would expect from a simple placebo effect* and has the attendant risks associated with inserting a microwave device in the prostatic urethra and destroying prostate tissue. Other reports from various investigators from 2002 to 2004 initially showed no improvement in CPPS using transurethral prostate needle radiofrequency heat ablation versus a sham procedure. One Taiwanese report on treatment of thirty-two patients using this technique in 2004 suggested a 68 percent improvement in a nonstandardized pain score.

PROSTATE AND PELVIC MASSAGE

Prostatic massage has been utilized by several generations of urologists, particularly prior to the advent of antibiotics. In a report from a Philippine study, repeated prostatic massages revealed occult organisms. This study received attention and popularity as a therapeutic benefit from massage expression of ductal contents that were not being emptied. This treatment may diminish prostatic pressure. The frequency of prostatic massage seems best when done twice weekly.

Dr. Daniel Shoskes proposed massage plus antibiotic treatment. His patients underwent prostatic massage plus antibiotics for two to eight weeks; 40 percent had complete resolution of symptoms, 20 percent had significant improvements, and 40 percent had no improvement. There was no correlation between inflammatory content and bacterial cultures. Our opinion, gained from research at Stanford as expressed in a review article from *Techniques in Urology*, favors repetitive massage of the prostate, not to empty the gland but rather to relieve pelvic tension and release myofascial trigger points. By our analysis, repeated prostate massage is a "blind approach" to treating the disorder, where occasionally the right trigger point or myofascial source is appropriately touched.

We continue to be extremely skeptical of the concept of occult bacteria that need to be "massaged out."

PELVIC FLOOR REHABILITATION

We are not the first doctors to have considered the kind of treatment we are describing in this book. As early as 1934, a few physicians understood that pelvic pain is related to tension or spasm of the pelvic muscles. George Thiele, M.D., a proctologist (who would now be referred to as a colorectal surgeon), developed a physical treatment for pelvic pain that he generally included under the name *coccygynia* (pain of the coccyx, or tailbone). In 1937 Thiele's findings were confirmed by Saul Shapiro, who referred to pain around the coccyx as the Thiele syndrome. In an article in 1963, Thiele reported on 324 patients who had pelvic pain in and around the rectum and anus and noted that there was no evidence of any disease of the coccyx or adjacent areas.

Thiele's contribution of applied massage to the levator ani and coccygeus muscles yielded remarkably good results. In some papers in the colorectal studies that followed, his treatment was referred to as Thiele massage. He reported that over 90 percent of people that he treated improved after such treatment. He was a pioneer in this area, and while he published his results for doctors in his field to consider, somehow his work disappeared and is rarely referred to in the literature on pelvic pain. The reason for this may be both economic and ideological. There is little economic incentive for colorectal surgeons to do Thiele massage. They do surgery, and they may not see massage of a patient's pelvic muscles as a good use of the surgeon's time.

Other specialists or physical therapists have been more likely to utilize this form of therapy for patients with CPPS. Mehrsheed Sinaki, M.D., was a physician at the Mayo Clinic in the department of physical medicine and rehabilitation throughout most of the 1970s. Doctor Sinaki reviewed the medical records of patients who had a diagnosis of pelvic pain in general, which at that time was more often referred to by the terms *piriformis syndrome, coccygodynia, levator ani spasm syndrome, proctalgia fugax,* or simply *rectal pain.* Absent were reports of urinary symptoms or of diagnoses such as prostatitis, interstitial cystitis, or some of the other conditions we include in this book.

Sinaki acknowledged that the conditions he examined were ob-
scured by many vague and chronic complaints. Furthermore, he found,
as we find today, that a general medical exam and routine laboratory and
x-ray exam were unremarkable. Sinaki believed that the definitive test
for the conditions he was reviewing was the digital-rectal examination
in which the doctor inserts a gloved lubricated finger into the rectum
to feel the state of the muscles. He observed, however, that the normal
digital-rectal examination was inadequate to assess the tenderness of the
muscles. Segura and other colleagues of Sinaki at the Mayo Clinic reiterated Sinaki's ideas in the *Journal of Urology* in 1979, noting that "patients with symptoms suggestive of prostatitis or prostatosis who do
not have pathogenic bacteria in the prostatic secretions may in fact not
have prostatic problems. The possibility of pelvic floor tension myalgia
should be considered."

We do not advocate biofeedback. We note, however, that a group
from Northwestern University Medical School in Chicago promotes the
use of biofeedback in pelvic floor reeducation as well as bladder training for this disorder. They recognize that pelvic floor tension myalgia
contributes to the symptoms. In 2000, J. Q. Clemens and colleagues
looked at a small group of nineteen men, average age of thirty-six years,
and treated them with this noninterventional process. The men not only
showed improvement in their urinary scores but also had a significant
decrease in their median pain scores, from 5 to 1 on a scale of 0 (no
symptoms) to 10 (worst symptoms). This was a preliminary study, but
it confirms that a formalized neuromuscular reeducation of the pelvic
floor muscles benefits some patients.

RESEARCH ON TRIGGER POINTS
AND PELVIC PAIN

Drs. David Hubbard and Gregory Berkoff of the Department of Neuro-
sciences at the University of California, San Diego, discovered that trigger points, which we usually find inside the pelvic floor of our patients,
show abnormal spontaneous electrical activity. Drs. Janet Travell and

David Simons, who introduced the concept of muscular trigger points and myofascial release, defined the standard by which trigger points could be identified:

1. Palpable and firm areas of muscle, usually referred to as the taut band
2. In the taut band, a little spot of great tenderness and sensitivity, especially upon the use of manual pressure
3. A pattern of sensation involving pain, sometimes in combination with tingling or numbness when this area is palpated digitally
4. What has been called a "local twitch" of this spot of tautness when the trigger point is pressed

Until the time of this study, trigger points could be identified only with a finger and there was no objective measure of the trigger point itself. The fact that trigger points could be identified only by individual palpation and not by objective measures left open their significance and even their reality. But Hubbard and Berkoff placed needle electrodes in the trigger points of the subjects of their study. They also placed needle electrodes immediately beside the trigger point within the same muscle. They connected the needle electrodes to an electromyograph (EMG), which is a very sensitive machine for measuring electrical activity. Electrical activity in muscle is considered to be a measure of its level of activity.

Their results were remarkable because they found a sustained level of increased electrical activity in the trigger point but no increased electrical activity in the tissue immediately beside the trigger point. They theorized that this prolonged increase in electrical activity becomes painful by affecting the spindle capsule. (The spindle capsule is a microscopic part of the muscle tissue that the authors speculated was affected by the increased electrical activity and was the source of pain.) This increased electrical activity was seen to be associated with the pain experienced subjectively, when the trigger point was pressed on or even when it was not.

We have found the presence of trigger points in a large majority of our patients who have pelvic pain and dysfunction. We typically are able to re-create the symptoms of patients we see when we press on these trigger points. We also find that when we complete a course of myofascial trigger point release, the trigger points usually mitigate or disappear along with the pain and exquisite sensitivity. Along with our own clinical experience, the findings in this study, in confirming objective and measurable activity specifically within the trigger point, offer compelling evidence that trigger points in the pelvic floor have central significance to a person's experience of pain in other chronic pelvic pain syndromes.

The reduction of trigger point sensitivity is often directly related to a subjective improvement in patient symptoms. Ralph Kruse and James Christiansen examined the temperature of the skin in the area to which pain was referred after a trigger point was palpated. Their study provides some objective basis for validating patients' reports of referred pain from a trigger point. They found that the area where a patient reported referred pain had a colder temperature than adjacent skin areas. It is assumed that the colder area was caused by a reduction in blood flow. Therefore, the area of referred pain being colder than the adjacent tissue supports the idea that ischemia (reduced blood flow) may be part of the pain and dysfunction we see in patients who have chronic pelvic pain syndrome.

In a conversation with Dr. Richard Gevirtz, who has done research on the relationship between trigger points and emotional reactivity, he shared with us that the impetus for the research that discovered increased electrical activity in trigger points in relationship to stress or anxiety originally came from Italian researchers and their work in the early and mid-1990s. They proposed that sympathetic nervous system activity directly affected skeletal muscle and particularly the spindle part of the muscle. Gevirtz and Hubbard showed that trigger point activity significantly increased when the subject experienced anxiety and that the trigger point activity decreased in the absence of emotional arousal. Needle electrodes monitored electrical activity in trigger points of subjects asked to do arithmetic calculations (a standard way in which researchers arouse anxiety). In considering the results of this study that connect anxiety and trigger point activity, we begin to make sense of the intimate relationship between stress and pelvic pain and dysfunction symptoms reported to us by many of our patients.

In our own work, we previously measured the level of muscle tension in the rectum and the vagina of patients who came to see us for pelvic pain and dysfunction. Men with prostatitis had an increased level of pelvic floor muscle tension. This level was reduced after they participated in the treatment program that has led to the current one. Dr. Howard Glazer at Cornell University in New York reported that men who had prostatodynia had higher-than-normal levels of rectal tension and that their resting level of tension was what he called "unstable" compared with normal subjects. Glazer has also consistently seen increased levels of vaginal tension in women who have vulvar pain. He sees a weakness in the strength of contraction of these women when asked to do Kegel exercises monitored by an electromyograph. The focus of Glazer's successful approach with women with vulvar pain has been to help them relax, strengthen, and stabilize their pelvic muscles.

THE *WISE-ANDERSON PROTOCOL*

After many years of treating patients with CPPS utilizing manual physical therapy as well as specific and extensive relaxation training, we determined that intensive or immersion therapy over several days was an ideal method to break long-term pain cycles and teach patients to care for themselves. Patients are evaluated by a urologist and then immerse themselves in daily physical therapy and *Extended Paradoxical Relaxation* training over a six-day period. We have conducted over 150 monthly sessions of this type with significant benefit to a large proportion of patients.

In our study, we hypothesized that palpation of certain myofascial trigger points would reproduce the pain sensations experienced by the patients. This was typically shown to be the case.

We reported a case series study of self-referred men with long-standing CPPS and attempted to describe the relationship between the locations of myofascial trigger points or restrictive muscular tissue, both internal and external to the pelvis, and the sites of pain initially described by the patients at the time of their evaluation. The same physical therapist performed manual myofascial tissue palpation on all subjects. A traditional palpation force of approximately for tender points (recommended for examination of fibromyalgia) was used for the assessment of pain. Pain was ranked as 0 (none) to 3+ (severe) for each area examined. Only categorical pain levels of 2+ or 3+ were counted as "Yes—pain is present," while scores of 0 or 1+ were counted as "No pain." Sets of muscles that typically reproduced pain sensation in specific locations referred from trigger points were chosen for the investigation.

The median age of the seventy-two men with CPPS in this analysis was forty years (range twenty to seventy-two; interquartile range thirty-two to forty-nine) with a median duration of symptoms of 44 months (range 4 to 408 months). The severity of symptoms at the time of the initial examination was measured by the pain Visual Analogue Scale (VAS) score and the NIH–Chronic Prostatitis Symptom Index (NIH-CPSI) score, with higher scores representing greater severity. The median VAS score was 5 out of 10 (range 1–9). The median NIH-CPSI overall score was 27 (possible maximum = 43) with a median pain domain score of 13 (possible maximum = 21), urinary complaints of 5 (possible maximum = 10), and quality of life score of 10.5 (possible maximum = 12). The median total number of self-reported locations of pain was four out of a possible seven predesignated sites. There was no correlation between pain score and total number of painful locations. However, we did find that tenderness in the puborectalis or pubococcygeus muscles or both was associated with a higher pain score.

Ninety percent of men stated that they felt pain associated with palpation of the puborectalis and/or pubococcygeus muscles.

Palpation of the puborectalis and/or pubococcygeus muscles elicited pain in the penis in 93 percent of the patients. At least two of the ten trigger points could elicit or refer pain to every one of the anatomical sites in a large number of patients, and every trigger point was able to reproduce pain in at least one site. The most reactive muscles were the rectus abdominis and external obliques; palpation of trigger points in these muscles elicited pain in four of the seven sites. Perineal pain was the most reproducible, being elicited by eight out of ten trigger points.

The frequency with which trigger point palpation referred pain to a patient's self-reported chronic pain location was remarkable. The odds ratio implied that these patients were thirty-two times more likely to have penile pain reproduced by the pubococcygeus muscle palpation than patients without penile pain. These physical examination findings may lead to greater understanding of pathogenic mechanisms and to more focused therapy. No asymptomatic men were examined as control subjects, so we are unable to compare how patients without CPPS would respond to these palpations. However, the purpose of this study was to examine patients with CPPS rather than to compare their responses to normal subjects'. Finally, it is difficult to objectively measure pain, so we relied on patients' self-reported responses. If a painful location was not reported during the initial history, we could not account for it in our later analyses.

HOW TO CONTACT US

For inquiries about the six-day immersion clinic or other information:

Email: ahip@sonic.net
Telephone: 1 (707) 332-1492 or (415) 550-6455
Website: www.pelvicpainhelp.com
Mail: National Center for Pelvic Pain Research
450 Sutter Street, Suite 1940
San Francisco, CA 94108

APPENDIX: STORIES OF PATIENTS IN THEIR OWN WORDS

The following stories are from reports of patients who over the years have been trained in the *Wise–Anderson Protocol*. We collected most of these stories earlier in our work. Most of these patients did not have the advantage of the internal trigger point wand, our 238-page post-clinic twenty-eight-day manual, Kindle video and audio tablet, or our new *Trigger Point Genie*. Despite the absence of these innovations, which have been game changers in our work, these stories speak volumes.

REPORT FROM A FIFTY-TWO-YEAR-OLD MALE PHYSICIAN (HE CAME TO THE CLINIC BEFORE THE INTERNAL TRIGGER POINT WAND)

I am a fifty-two-year-old internist (family doctor for adults) with a busy practice in Los Angeles and the married father of two small children. I was completely caught off guard in 2005 by the symptoms of deep pelvic/perineal pain that remained intermittent for a month. The pain began to wake me up at night . . . I feared I might have cancer and had difficulty sitting. Advil didn't help.

I had back xrays, MRIs, laboratory studies, prostate exams: all normal. I became depressed, was sleep disturbed, despite Ambien, and was in constant pain and exhausted. The urologist said I had chronic prostatitis and suggested frequent hot baths and ejaculations and a trial of Flomax, Hytrin, Cardura, or Uroxatral, Proscar, or Avodart . . . I developed side effects and stopped taking those medications. I began crying intermittently, making life difficult at home and at work. In addition, I had urinary frequency every hour, making it difficult to see patients. I understood why people with such severe medical problems contemplated suicide. Several urologists suggested drinking a large volume of liquid, taking quercetin, and increasing sexual activity—nothing helped . . . I was in a very bad way. My wife started to check out the Internet to treat "chronic prostatitis." She read about the *Wise-Anderson Protocol* and pointed out that my symptoms were almost exactly what Dr. Wise discussed. My life revolved around pain, urinary frequency, constipation, and increasing depression. I found no joy in anything, including my children. It was now November 2005 and my wife finally coaxed me into calling Dr. Wise to see if he could offer any help. I was pretty skeptical. Effective treatments for diseases are not secret, and if they are successful everybody realizes it sooner or later. The urologists I had consulted would have the same information—right?

I drove out the first morning to Dr. Wise's compound expecting nothing. . . . I met the other dozen or so patients with similar symptoms—many of them had had symptoms for years! We spent long days together doing group relaxation, learning stretches, and having Trigger Point Release by Tim Sawyer. By the end of the first day I noticed that somehow the need to urinate had lessened slightly and that I didn't have to always use the bathroom during these sessions. I noticed that the pain itself would diminish (although at first just temporarily) after the trigger point release sessions.

I was still symptomatic that first evening but had a glimmer of hope.

I woke up on the third morning and had my first normal bowel movement in months. This is not normally reason for celebration, but I was feeling increasingly hopeful. I experienced progressive improvement over the ensuing days of the program, with diminution of all of the symptoms I had been experiencing. The symptoms did wax and wane, and I was hopeful when they improved but depressed when they returned. I completely stopped taking my meds . . . I concluded that these drugs play absolutely no role in this disorder.

My pain, constipation, urinary frequency, and, most important, mood had dramatically improved. I distinctly remember sitting in the airplane terminal in Oakland going back to Los Angeles and feeling completely euphoric! I was totally asymptomatic! I did not have to use the bathroom even once from Oakland to Los Angeles (probably a total of 3 hours overall). That was the longest voiding interval I had in probably 3 to 4 months.

Alas, much as Dr. Wise predicted, my euphoria and lack of symptoms were not to last. When I arrived back in Los Angeles and went back to the stress of my career and life, the symptoms came back over about a week's time, although not to the extent they were before the Stanford Protocol clinic.

The symptoms again improved over the next several months . . . I was feeling hopeful, although there were continued exacerbations and remission of my symptoms. I had improved significantly but now hoped for complete resolution of my symptoms. I asked my physical therapist (whom I had known and used for years for a variety of minor musculo-skeletal conditions) if he would be willing to learn the technique. I gave him a copy of *A Headache in the Pelvis*. After several sessions he was able to perform the Trigger Point Release effectively.

With the addition of this to my daily stretching and 2 to 3 times weekly relaxation tapes, I have had minimal symptoms since about the beginning of May 2006. I attribute all of the success to the method that Dr. Wise and his colleagues have worked out. I take no medication whatsoever right now and have no constipation, urinary frequency, and virtually no pain. I also can sit in any chair I want without a cushion (I had to take a cushion to restaurants when my symptoms were at their worst).

As a physician I am almost shocked about the lack of knowledge and the ridiculous suggestions by the urologists I had consulted. I mentioned earlier the recommendation to drink beer. Some of the other sexual recommendations are almost comical, such as "not holding back" during sex and having sex exactly three times per week. To their credit, they didn't seem offended when I offered to give them a copy of Dr. Wise's book. As Dr. Wise points out in his book, there are a multitude of reasons that urologists are not enlightened about this disorder, which is indeed unfortunate as it is one of the most common disorders for which urologists are consulted.

REPORT FROM A TWENTY-SEVEN-YEAR-OLD BUSINESSMAN

My pelvic pain started at the left tip of my penis. I went to over twenty doctors, checked myself into the hospital emergency room, did a CT scan, ultrasounds, and many other schemes to find the cause of this pain. Gradually my pain spread, and sitting, sleeping, walking, and every part of living was painful. Through my research on the Internet I believed I may have pudendal nerve entrapment. I had a pudendal nerve latency test. It came back positive, showing irregular reactions from my pudendal nerve.

PNE was a term that horrified me. The information on the Internet indicated that given my test results I would never be able to have pain-free sex, sitting would always be painful, and as time went on I would get worse. I read online that some people were trying new physical therapy techniques to improve their condition. I found a local therapist and started to work with her. I started to feel slightly better with internal trigger point releases. However, despite the temporary relief, I always found the pain returning.

She gave me a bunch of books to read, one of them being *A Headache in the Pelvis*. I was overwhelmed that there was a book out there that described my condition in full detail. I was finally empowered to take control of my condition. I completely dedicated my life to healing. I would spend anywhere from four to eight hours per day doing *Paradoxical Relaxation,* stretches, and skin rolling, or jog and sit in the hot tub. I actually invested in a hot tub and a treadmill. That's how dedicated I was.

Within four months I was completely pain free. Once I complied with the protocol 100 percent, I felt 100 percent better. . . . without the protocol, I probably would have been in physical and mental pain forever.

REPORT FROM A FORTY-ONE-YEAR-OLD FEMALE EXECUTIVE

It all started at a Halloween party in 2009, where my boyfriend's band was playing. My abdominal pains were so intense that I left the party before the band even started. I visited my general practitioner, who ordered a battery of tests. In the end, I was diagnosed with *H. pylori*. I was prescribed a ten-day course of intense antibiotics . . . I stuck with the program and the *H. pylori* infection was resolved.

A month after I finished the antibiotics, on a Saturday night, I started having symptoms of a UTI. The next day, Sunday, was perhaps the most painful day of my life. I was doubled over in pain the whole day . . .

My practitioners at the integrated clinic said it was likely that I had interstitial cystitis, but that the procedure for diagnosis, cystoscopy, often causes confounding bladder problems. Although it turned out that I didn't have IC, at least my practitioners didn't exacerbate my situation, as is the case for so many other CPPS patients. I clung to this bit of information—that my acupuncturist healed herself—as I began my search for a cure. If she could do it, then so could I.

I restricted my diet, lost 20 pounds, and socially withdrew. Eventually I found a physical therapist and had drastically reduced pain the day after I saw her. She lent me her copy of *A Headache in the Pelvis* and I read it in a single sitting. These guys, Drs. Wise and Anderson, got it.

I went to the clinic in August 2010 and my life will never be the same. I went knowing that physical therapy already worked for me, and I was looking forward to learning the self-treatment trigger point techniques.

The rest of clinic was a dream. It was such a relief to be in a room full of people who understood the frustration of living with chronic pelvic pain, and it was empowering to learn the recovery techniques from Dr. Wise and Tim.

After clinic, my symptoms diminished abruptly. Within two months, I felt normal on a fairly regular basis. I started testing foods I hadn't eaten in months, and to my delight I tolerated them. I still have occasional flares, but they're much milder.

The relaxation tapes have cured me from my pelvic pain and have given me a tool to get rid of any tension and anxiety. I can't thank them enough for that!

REPORT FROM A FORTY-FOUR-YEAR-OLD MALE HEDGE FUND MANAGER

I have been meaning to write you a note for some time. I have benefited greatly from your program, and my symptoms have decreased to the level of being insignificant. While this has probably been the single worst year of my career and I have lost significant amounts of money in my business (I manage a hedge fund), my pelvic pain has disappeared using your protocol.

REPORT FROM A FORTY-SEVEN-YEAR-OLD WOMAN

After the clinic, my symptoms diminished abruptly. Within two months, I picked up the second edition of this book and couldn't put it down. For once someone understood; it got straight to the heart of the matter.

After thirty years of mild pain followed by seven years of chronic and severely debilitating pain, I knew I was on the right path. It had felt for years that I was in emotional solitary confinement, unable to share the extent of the pain with anyone who could really know what I was talking about. However, many years on and £30,000 later, I had some of the jigsaw pieces and had started to make some progress toward full health, but it wasn't until I read this book that the full picture emerged.

I arrived in California and met fourteen men and women with the one common denominator of pelvic pain and its debilitating effects on life.

Every day of the protocol, we each had a session with Tim Sawyer, the protocol's chief physical therapist. And yet what a gift he gave all of us. He taught us to find trigger points, those knotty sore areas of muscle that triggered pain elsewhere.

Five days later I left Santa Rosa feeling renewed in spirit and knowing that I was on a journey that would lead to a full recovery. Eleven months after my visit I am 90 percent better.

You can't beat this pain by trying, striving, or driving for a cure. You have to be with it, allow it, almost befriend it, and then slowly it subsides; that's the amazing paradox.

REPORT FROM A TWENTY-FIVE-YEAR-OLD MALE ATTORNEY

In 2001, when I was twenty-three years old, I was walking to class and started to feel a pain at the tip of my penis. The doctor found no infection, and referred me to a urologist. The urologist also found no infection and said that there was nothing wrong with me. In a way, I believed him wholeheartedly, and even wanted to.

For over a year, I simply put up with the pain. Sometimes the pain wasn't that bad, sometimes it was terribly annoying. I developed other symptoms: pain in the urethra during ejaculation and, afterward, frequency and urgency related to urination. However, the severity of my symptoms always stayed manageable, and I carried on without telling a soul about my symptoms.

As I graduated from professional school and started my working life, my pain started to get worse. I was in a high-stress job, and my pain began to spread into my legs, perineum, hips, and back. From 2001 until 2004 (before I discovered the Stanford Protocol [*Wise-Anderson Protocol*]), I went to several different urologists, and basically I got the same treatment as most other men diagnosed with prostatitis: antibiotics, anti-inflammatories, and even anti-depressants for "psychosomatic" pain. Nothing helped.

Finally, my pain exploded, and I could no longer carry on my routine. I was in so much distress. I hurt 24/7, and I fell into severe depression. I truly believed my life was over. I had a dark night of the soul.

Then I found *A Headache in the Pelvis* on the Internet. I read it and it described perfectly what I was experiencing. I discovered my entire body, and especially my pelvis, was riddled with trigger points. Immediately I went to California and attended one of the clinics. I learned Paradoxical Relaxation from Dr. Wise and the basics of trigger point therapy from Tim Sawyer, both internally and externally. I immediately felt better, but knew that I had a very long way to go before I could consistently reduce my symptoms.

During these past two years that I have been practicing the Stanford Protocol [the *Wise-Anderson Protocol*], there have been many ups and downs. I have continued to improve. In fact, the setbacks for me were not that I physically felt any worse, but rather that I had to work through my anger about no one ever teaching these wonderful truths about my muscles to me, and how it related to the central nervous system. I was mad that I had not been raised on the teachings in *A Headache in the Pelvis*.

My pelvic musculature is, I would say, about 97 percent healed, and I know over the course of the next year it will slowly dissolve.

REPORT FROM A THIRTY-NINE-YEAR-OLD WOMAN

I struggled with pain during intercourse since I lost my virginity at age seventeen. It was extremely painful that first time and continued to be so for nearly twenty years. For many years, I had no idea that it wasn't supposed to hurt. I was in major denial, not wanting to face this very personal and sensitive subject.

A few months later, my husband and I visited Dr. Wise's clinic in Sebastopol. After learning and doing the physical therapy and breathing exercises for just a few weeks, we had nearly pain-free sex, and I got pregnant again! I continued with the breathing exercises and physical therapy daily for the following nine months. I credit the relaxation I achieved from these exercises with helping me have a vaginal birth with no drugs whatsoever (this was only twelve months after a drug-filled C-section!). The vaginal birth has made a tremendous difference for me. I oftentimes now have no pain or discomfort during intercourse. I hope that continuing with Dr. Wise's protocol will make me 100 percent pain-free in the near future.

Dr. Wise's protocol is not an easy fix. It takes time, patience, and perseverance. It has helped me be more comfortable with my own body and in relating sexually to my husband with more comfort, pleasure, and, therefore, intimacy.

REPORT FROM AN EIGHTY-ONE-YEAR-OLD WOMAN (WITHOUT THE USE OF THE INTERNAL TRIGGER POINT WAND)

You may very well have forgotten me, since we have not communicated by phone since the spring of 2004. It is about time that I reported to you on my progress.

With the recommendation of Dr. Jeannette Potts, Cleveland Clinic, you agreed to give me instruction by phone. I did the tape and exercises every day and the therapeutic massage nearly every week until the end of 2007. My whole mindset has changed. The more knowledge I gained, the more my body calmed down. My lifelong pattern of trying to be perfect has eased considerably. Looking back over the years I can see the tension I created for myself. And I finally admitted that I was the one who had to change and take the time to retrain myself. And it has taken time.

I have been free of pain for over five months. This is totally wonderful, since I began this situation in 1988. I continue to do the tapes and exercises several times a week, and from time to time read a few pages of your book. These things seem to be necessary to maintain my good health. Now that I am approaching eighty-one(!) there will hopefully be a few more good years!

REPORT FROM A TWENTY-TWO-YEAR-OLD MALE (PRIOR TO THE AVAILABILITY OF THE INTERNAL TRIGGER POINT WAND)

I suffered from prostatitis/CPPS for three years, and my life became absolutely miserable. I received four different diagnoses from four urologists, tried over twenty prescription medications, vitamins, and herbs, and underwent several very uncomfortable and expensive procedures, all of which did hardly anything to help my symptoms, which had slowly been increasing in intensity over time. Using the protocol described in *A Headache in the Pelvis,* I slowly began to heal myself without any medication. Six months later my symptoms diminished significantly, and nine months later I felt I was healed. It is now two and a half years after I first started to practice these methods, and I feel that I have been freed of this horrific condition.

REPORT FROM A MALE PATIENT AFTER PRACTICING THE PROTOCOL FOR EIGHT MONTHS (PRIOR TO AVAILABILITY OF INTERNAL TRIGGER POINT WAND)

I am a thirty-five-year-old male who, until recently, suffered from chronic prostatitis for over fifteen years. I am writing to share my experience in the hope that someone else currently suffering from my predicament can heal as I have.

Starting at about age eighteen, I began to notice symptoms of high urinary frequency and a great sense of urgency when I felt the need to urinate. By the time I was twenty-four, the symptoms reached the point where I was uncomfortable much of the day.

I went to see multiple doctors, including several urologists diagnosing me from chronic prostatitis to a narrow bladder neck. I took alpha blockers, which were no help.

I always sat on the aisle row of a movie theater, would map out the restrooms upon first entering an unfamiliar place, felt the urge to urinate every hour during the day, and experienced poor sleep quality.

In October 2002, the inconvenient and annoying symptoms of my condition turned into a persistent pain. When urinating no longer relieved me in and around my urethra, my bladder, and my prostate, I was given a diagnosis of "chronic prostatitis." I started taking antibiotics, alpha blockers, Ambien to sleep at night, muscle relaxants, and anti-inflammatory drugs. None of these helped.

I began missing work, spent entire days in tears, suffered from panic attacks, and visited the emergency room. I started to avoid people as much as possible.

I had an MBA from Harvard Business School. I had a great job, loving wife, and two children. I had a strong relationship with God. Yet, I couldn't see how I was going to survive. I didn't see how I could possibly maintain my job . . . Sex was out of the question because it just exacerbated the symptoms. I would have gladly given up all my money and material possessions to be cured of the acute pain that plagued my every moment.

I learned about the work of Drs. Wise and Anderson. Contrary to many other approaches I read about on the Internet, their approach appealed to me because it had a fundamental basis that did not entail pharmaceuticals or surgery.

Within a week after the clinic, I was much better.

It has now been eight months since I started this program. I have had to dedicate significant time to this effort. I feel like a miracle has been granted to me. My urinary frequency has dropped to only once per night and once per two hours, at most, during the day. I feel little, if any, pain. I feel almost no pain following sex. I am better than I have been in over fifteen years!

MALE RECOVERY WITH NO PHYSICAL THERAPY OR FORMAL RELAXATION TRAINING

(While most patients require both Paradoxical Relaxation training and intrapelvic Trigger Point Release, we have received emails from people reporting that their symptoms improved after the reading of our book and hearing of a possible solution to their difficulty. Here is the story of a patient like this.)

I first experienced prostatitis when I was around twenty-three. It would not go away, and it had this rather strange tendency to occasionally migrate. The discomfort generally didn't go away. After about eight years, I had pretty much resigned myself to living with that condition indefinitely, which was not a rosy picture at all.

I came across the findings of Dr. Wise. I was struck by two things. It seemed he had a handle on what was going on . . . The second thing was the real breakthrough: the possibility that the ultimate source of this discomfort was not any infection, not any structural abnormality, but simply TENSION, muscular tightness that restricted the entire area that was affected.

To make a long story short, this basic insight was nothing less than a breakthrough for me. Within about a six-month period, after simply learning about what was really going on, miraculously, the pain went away! I am now free of prostatitis.

TWENTY-YEAR-OLD MALE

I was twenty years old when my symptoms started with a vengeance . . . in constant pain, with a deep ache in my pelvis, and the urge to urinate all day and night. For months I don't think I slept longer than an hour at a time (usually intervals of twenty to forty minutes) even with sleeping aids.

However, since reading this book, being fortunate enough to attend the clinic, and actively applying the methods I learned, I have made tremendous improvement. My symptoms have decreased, in a conservative estimate, by 75 percent, and, sometimes, I am pain free. Things I could have only dreamed of when this torture started. So for those who despair, as I once did, there is hope, and for many I believe that hope lies with actively practicing the methods that are taught within this book.

MALE PATIENT REPORT AFTER PRACTICING PROTOCOL FOR TWO YEARS (PRIOR TO AVAILABILITY OF THE INTERNAL TRIGGER POINT WAND)

In October 2000 I had a vasectomy. I began to experience severe pains in my testicles, which forced me to give up employment. For several months I was unable to do much more than stay in bed. In addition to the pain, I was unable to ejaculate.

I was given large doses of opiates, 36 mg of Hydromorph Contin per day, which did nothing for the underlying condition. In November 2001, I came upon "The New Theory That Prostatitis Is a Tension Disorder." I spoke to Dr. Wise a number of times on the phone, and in December 2001 I went to California. I was seen by Dr. Rodney Anderson, a urologist, and Tim Sawyer, a physiotherapist. My wife accompanied me on the visit and learned the technique of myofascial release inside the pelvic floor from Tim Sawyer, and I began daily relaxation training.

By the late months of 2002, I was taking only 1 mg of hydrocodone per day. Since January 2003 I have taken no painkillers on a regular basis. I visited Dr. Wise and Tim Sawyer again in March 2003. Tim was able to confirm a significant loosening inside the pelvic floor. I continue to feel some pain every day, but rarely is the pain severe enough to take any opiate. The degree of pain from day to day varies a great deal. Some days are entirely pain-free except for occasional discomfort in the pelvic area; some days involve pain for longer periods and more intensity. There is usually some pain during and after sexual intercourse, but ejaculations are normal.

In general I would say I am pain free about three-quarters to seven-eighths of the time.

MALE PATIENT REPORT AFTER PRACTICING PROTOCOL FOR FOUR YEARS (PRIOR TO AVAILABILITY OF INTERNAL TRIGGER POINT WAND)

Beginning in about 1992 (age twenty-seven), I experienced occasional pelvic pain. I am a military lawyer, and when I was stationed overseas from 1994 to 1996, the pain became progressively worse, including a low urine flow and occasional sharp rectal pain.

I was diagnosed with chronic prostatitis. In 1997 I experienced these symptoms on and off. In 1998, the symptoms became worse. Despite no evidence of infection, I was prescribed ciprofloxacin 500 for about seventy-five days for chronic prostatitis.

Fortunately, the military urologist had heard a paper delivered by Dr. Rodney Anderson.

Over the course of my year of training in progressive (paradoxical) relaxation, I learned to totally relax my mind and body. When I received myofascial release therapy from a physical therapist prescribed by Dr. Wise, I could actually feel when the tension inside was released by stretching the tissue.

In the last four years, I have integrated this relaxation method into my life. I try to make time for one complete session of progressive (paradoxical) relaxation session each day, but in my current position I cannot always do so.

Usually I have no pelvic pain, a strong urine flow, and a sense that my bladder is emptied after urination. Usually the pain is nonexistent, but will fairly rarely be present at a low level if I become very stressed or busy at work. This stands in stark contrast to before I began the protocol when the pain was there all the time and occasionally severe.

This treatment and protocol have changed my life.

REPORT FROM A MOTHER OF A TWENTY-YEAR-OLD MAN

My twenty-year-old son took your seminar last June. I just wanted to thank all of you for giving him the tools to get his life back. Today he just ran out of the house to go to the beach with friends. He teaches sailing to young people at a local club and attends college in NYC. He uses the meditation tapes and other exercises, but his episodes of discomfort are farther and farther apart.

REPORT FROM A THIRTY-NINE-YEAR-OLD WOMAN WHO GAVE BIRTH

I wanted to drop you a line to let you know that I gave birth to a healthy baby boy on 6/1/2011. He came just slightly early (twelve days) but thankfully full-term. He was born via C-section, which turns out was the right thing for me (my firstborn was delivered naturally with much trauma to my pelvic floor). I am recovering very well from surgery and have not had any flare-ups of pelvic pain. In fact, my pain level declined significantly during pregnancy after I was put on bed rest at thirty weeks due to a shortened cervix.

I want to thank you for your support during a trying time. I was really scared once my flare-up started, but luckily as intense as the pain was, it had no impact on the progress of my pregnancy.

I hope I can be a source of hope for women with my condition who plan to have children. So far, I haven't resumed internal work yet because I'm still not six weeks postpartum (when pelvic rest is prescribed).

With all honesty I can say that without the *Wise-Anderson Protocol*, I may not have had the courage to try again for another baby.

REPORT FROM A TWENTY-YEAR-OLD MAN

Today I am very fit and healthy, I exercise daily, and I take no drugs. Today I did a small video review to show my experience and how I managed to get my health back. I will be forever grateful for your help, and it is a pleasure to have been able to know you. Hopefully someday we will meet again.

MALE PATIENT REPORT AFTER FIVE YEARS OF PRACTICING PROTOCOL (PRIOR TO AVAILABILITY OF THE INTERNAL TRIGGER POINT WAND)

In late September 1997, two years after retiring, I started having problems with urination . . . The doctor prescribed an antibiotic and referred me to a urologist. The urologist prescribed traditional treatment for prostate infection, including antibiotic and ibuprofen. . . . No help.

The symptoms were ruining my life, and, at times, I was depressed. I was losing weight and there didn't seem to be any light at the end of the tunnel.

A close friend got me an appointment in mid-December 1997 with Dr. Tom Stamey, the pioneer of urology at Stanford University, department of urology. Stamey determined in one hour that I had no evidence of infection and referred me to Rodney Anderson.

Dr. Anderson had me see a physical therapist that specialized in myofascial pelvic floor muscle pain relief. Dr. Wise started to teach me Paradoxical Relaxation. Gradually, I started to make progress. One day, a few months after starting his therapy, I asked him how long it would take to perfect his technique. He hesitated for a while, but finally said "about two years."

My progress steadily got better and after a year I was 80 percent better. After two years I felt like I had reduced my symptoms by 90 percent.

It is now about five years since I first started treatment with Drs. Anderson and Wise. I feel that my symptoms are 99 percent gone.

REPORT FROM A FORTY-FOUR-YEAR-OLD MALE PHYSICIAN

I first met Dr. Wise at age forty-four after a fifteen-year history of constant urinary urgency, suprapubic discomfort, and constipation, which was exacerbated by any exercise requiring sitting in a squatted position. Sex could worsen my symptoms, in addition to ill-fitting seats. I took multiple antibiotics, Hytrin, Elavil, and Flomax without improvement. I was told that I had mild interstitial cystitis. Overall I believe there is a 90 percent plus improvement for me, and after fifteen-plus years of pelvic pain, I am very grateful.

REPORT FROM A FIFTY-FOUR-YEAR-OLD WOMAN

The *Wise-Anderson Protocol* has been a godsend for me. I suffered for over thirty years with disabling pelvic pain and tried every available medical and alternative treatment without success. After using the *Wise-Anderson Protocol* for less than a year now, I am for the first time on my way to a pain-free life.

REPORT FROM A FIFTEEN-YEAR-OLD ATHLETIC MALE

When my fifteen-year-old athletic son was in excruciating pain and no one could offer help, Dr. Wise's book and program was literally a lifesaver. I make it a point to speak to every health care provider about this book and program, just in case this information can help someone suffering as my son was.

REPORT FROM A SIXTY-YEAR-YEAR-OLD FEMALE LAWYER

When I attended the seminar in 2006, I had spent four frustrating years going from expert to expert in the Northeast medical community. Each physician had a different idea of what my problem was and how to treat it. I was literally at my wit's end and had been unable to work for a month because I was in so much pain. I found Dr. Wise and his associates by researching my symptoms online and buying and reading his book and contacting him. His phone call to me was the first sign of relief I had had. After attending the workshop, learning, and practicing Paradoxical Relaxation, and seeing physical therapists he recommended, I was able to recover and return to work. I have had a few flare-ups over the ten years since, but I know how to help myself and what works for me. I am very grateful.

ACKNOWLEDGMENTS

We wish to express our gratitude to the following individuals who have helped and inspired us in the writing of this book: Elaine Orenberg Anderson, Julie Smolin, John Moses, Harold Wise, Erik Peper, Ruth Dreier, Ramana Maharshi, Jean Klein, Kathy Harris, Helen Wise, Frederick Perls, Jim Simkin, Martin Schwartz, Alan Leveton, Ann Armstrong, Ann Dreyfuss, Leo Zeff, Walter Kaufmann, Milton Rosenberg. Special thanks to Marilyn Freedman for her help with the sections on pelvic pain and childbirth and anorectal disorders. We express our deep appreciation for the seminal work of Dr. Edmund Jacobson in Progressive Relaxation and to Drs. Janet Travell and David Simons for their work in trigger point release. We are particularly indebted to Tim Sawyer, PT, for his great skill, talent, and experience in trigger point release related to pelvic pain; he has been our senior consultant in physical therapy in our work when we were at Stanford and is the architect of the *Wise-Anderson Protocol* physical therapy methodology.

INDEX

Page numbers in *italics* refer to illustrations.

ABOUT THE AUTHORS

David Wise, Ph.D., worked with Stanford urologist Dr. Rodney Anderson over an eight-year period in treating men and women who suffered from pelvic pain and urinary and sexual dysfunction who were given a variety of diagnoses with what is now called the Wise-Anderson Protocol. Wise is a psychologist in California and his research interests are in behavioral medicine and autonomic self-regulation.

Rodney U. Anderson, M.D., FACS, is Professor of Urology (Emeritus-active) at Stanford University School of Medicine. His subspecialty clinical expertise is neuro-urology and female urology. His focus has been on chronic pelvic pain syndromes, pelvic floor dysfunction, interstitial cystitis, benign prostatic hyperplasia, urinary incontinence, urinary retention, spinal cord injuries, spina bifida, multiple sclerosis, Parkinsonism, and stroke. He has also directed a clinic devoted to the problem of female sexual dysfunction. He continues to be actively engaged in clinical research at Stanford on the *Wise-Anderson Protocol* and other research.